Compression and Chronic Wound Management

Raj Mani · Kittipan Rerkasem
Harikrishna K. R. Nair · Vijay Shukla
Editors

Compression and Chronic Wound Management

Springer

Editors
Raj Mani
University of Southampton Hospital
Southampton
Hampshire
UK

Kittipan Rerkasem
Maharaj Naikom Hospital
Chiang Mai University
Chiang Mai
Thailand

Harikrishna K. R. Nair
Hospital Kuala Lumpur
Kuala Lumpur
Malaysia

Vijay Shukla
Department of General Surgery
Banaras Hindu University
Varanasi
Uttar Pradesh
India

ISBN 978-3-030-01194-9 ISBN 978-3-030-01195-6 (eBook)
https://doi.org/10.1007/978-3-030-01195-6

Library of Congress Control Number: 2018964061

This Springer imprint is published by the registered company Springer Nature Switzerland AG
The registered company address is: Gewerbestrasse 11, 6330 Cham, Switzerland

Preface

Compression and Chronic Wounds

Some decades ago, when the four-layer elasticated bandage (then called the Charing Cross bandage) was developed for treating venous leg ulcers, it seemed the answer to a maiden's prayer. It was possible to deliver better pressures, it seemed like the bandages would hold up better and we expected improved healing rates. Of course, our nurses needed specific training, and then there was the matter of finding additional costs associated with the bandages. Good data were gathered reliably. We understood healing rates in our own areas, learnt that bulky bandages interfere with wearing shoes and, perhaps the most important of all, that replicating a perfect bandage is an art form. During this period, there was much innovation of bandaging systems: developments of bandages with more tension, with imprinted figures to guide the hand that wrapped the bandage around legs, the short-stretch bandage and so on. The knowledge that pressure beneath the bandage varies with position and ambulation and pressure-measuring sensors also appeared. A lot of this was grist to the mill for our admired friend and colleague Hugo Partsch who has emphasised the importance of measuring calf circumference and the level (B1 point) on the calf where it should be done. With all this, it continues to be reasonable to expect that compression bandaging will benefit some 50% of the population with chronic wounds. So, what becomes of the remainder? What about patients who are wheelchair bound? And others who live in the upper floors of apartments with no lifts—how would they get to a clinic to be treated with compression dressings? And above all what about those with venous disease or lymphoedema? How could we reasonably advise them to wear bandages/garments over their legs in environments where the mercury rarely drops below 30 °C during the day? These were arguments had by the four of us when we met in some meeting or other. And so, the idea was born to write this book.

During all this period, devices have been innovated and tried and the findings are clear. Mechanical compression does improve venous return. But will wounds heal? Do you select a wound for a device? When is its use optimally indicated?

Surgery is a vital albeit another track. Based on the latest developments and evidence, surgical management of superficial vein incompetence in Asian societies (with younger demographics), with expectations of wound healing and low recurrence, may have a great deal to offer to such patients.

Going back to the whole picture, devices are recent on the scene. There is a need for a new paradigm that brings together surgery with devices and compression bandaging. The legend of Cinderella was interesting to hear as a child: in a real world, one shoe will not fit all. If you are wondering about costs, what is the true value of device or drug? Surely it must depend on getting it to the number who need it. This book reinforces the importance of compression to treat venous disease and lymphoedema. It discusses new devices and their associated benefits. The book also offers glimpses into the use of traditional medicine systems (Ayurvedic and Chinese) to treat lymphoedema and chronic wounds.

Southampton, Hampshire, UK — Raj Mani
Varanasi, Uttar Pradesh, India — Vijay Shukla
Chiang Mai, Thailand — Kittipan Rerkasem
Kuala Lumpur, Malaysia — Harikrishna K. R. Nair
July 2018

Contents

Contributors

Naseer Ahmad Manchester University Foundation Trust, Manchester, UK

Translational Medicine, University of Manchester, Manchester, UK

Greater Manchester and East Cheshire Strategic Clinical Network, Manchester, UK

Frank Lee Bowling Manchester University Foundation Trust, Manchester, UK

Translational Medicine, University of Manchester, Manchester, UK

Diabetes Task Force Lead, World Health Organization, Geneva, Switzerland

Andrew Ross Cameron The University of Queensland, St Lucia, QLD, Australia

Christine Faure-Chazelles Montpellier University Hospital, Montpellier Cedex, France

Mieke Flour Dermatology, University Hospitals Leuven, Leuven, Belgium

Georgina Gethin National University of Ireland Galway, Galway, Ireland

Joon Pio (Jp) Hong Department of Plastic and Reconstructive Surgery, Asan Medical Center, University of Ulsan College of Medicine, Seoul, South Korea

Yao Huang Wound Healing Center at Emergency Department, Ninth People's Hospital, Shanghai Jiao Tong University School of Medicine, Shanghai, China

Raj Mani Faculty of Medicine, Academic Division of Human Development & Health, University of Southampton, Southampton, UK

Faculty of Medicine, Chiang Mai University, Chiang Mai, Thailand

Shanghai Jiao Tong University School of Medicine, Shanghai, China

Ravi Mani Brighton and Sussex Medical School, University of Brighton, Brighton, UK

Faculty of Medicine, Chiang Mai University, Chiang Mai, Thailand

Faculty of Medicine, Academic Division of Human Development & Health, University of Southampton, Southampton, UK

Marguerite Guillot Masanovic Montpellier University Hospital, Montpellier Cedex, France

Harikrishna K. R. Nair Wound Care Unit, Department of Internal Medicine, Kuala Lumpur Hospital, Kuala Lumpur, Malaysia

Department of Surgery, Institute of Medical Sciences, Banares Hindu University, Varanasi, Uttar Pradesh, India

S. R. Narahari Institute of Applied Dermatology, Kasaragod, Kerala, India

Pengwen Ni Wound Healing Center at Emergency Department, Ninth People's Hospital, Shanghai Jiao Tong University School of Medicine, Shanghai, China

Saritphat Orrapin Faculty of Medicine, Division of Vascular and Endovascular Surgery, Department of Surgery, Thammasat University Hospital, Thammasat University, Pathum Thani, Thailand

Hugo Partsch Medical University of Vienna, Vienna, Austria

K. S. Prasanna Institute of Applied Dermatology, Kasaragod, Kerala, India

Kittipan Rerkasem Faculty of Medicine, Division of Vascular and Endovascular Surgery, Department of Surgery, Chiang Mai University, Chiang Mai, Thailand

Department of Surgery, NCD Centre of Excellence, Chiang Mai University, Chiang Mai, Thailand

Mark C. Richardson University of Southampton, Southampton, UK

Vijay K. Shukla Department of General Surgery, Institute of Medical Sciences, Banaras Hindu University, Varanasi, Uttar Pradesh, India

Boonying Siribumrungwong Faculty of Medicine, Division of Vascular and Endovascular Surgery, Department of Surgery, Thammasat University Hospital, Thammasat University, Pathum Thani, Thailand

Vivek Srivastava Department of General Surgery, Institute of Medical Sciences, Banaras Hindu University, Varanasi, Uttar Pradesh, India

Hyunsuk Peter Suh Department of Plastic and Reconstructive Surgery, Asan Medical Center, University of Ulsan College of Medicine, Seoul, South Korea

Luc Téot Montpellier University Hospital, Montpellier Cedex, France

Qi Wang Wound Healing Center at Emergency Department, Ninth People's Hospital, Shanghai Jiao Tong University School of Medicine, Shanghai, China

Yunfei Wang LongHua Hospital, Shanghai University of Traditional Chinese Medicine, Shanghai, China

Xian Xiao Wound Healing Center at Emergency Department, Ninth People's Hospital, Shanghai Jiao Tong University School of Medicine, Shanghai, China

Ting Xie Wound Healing Center at Emergency Department, Ninth People's Hospital, Shanghai Jiao Tong University School of Medicine, Shanghai, China

Chapter 1
The Public Health Burden of Chronic Wounds Needs a Whole Systems Approach

Naseer Ahmad, Frank Lee Bowling, and Raj Mani

Abstract The burden of chronic wounds is rising and therefore significant on both individuals and society. Whilst the mainstay of leg ulcer care is compression, the provision of this service is actually sporadic. This inequity is partly responsible for varying outcomes of care. In order to improve outcomes, a detailed understanding of the patient journey through a 'whole systems analysis' is required. Here, a detailed analysis of the processes and organisations the patient comes into contact with are understood and optimised to improve outcome.

Keywords Whole systems analysis · Patient journey · Public health · Inequality

Chronic wounds represent a significant burden to individuals and to societies at large. This is because the costs of managing these wounds are increasing on account of the inflation of health-related costs, rising longevity and increasing prevalence of diabetes as well as peripheral arterial disease. The causes of these wounds are multifactorial and not confined to the disease risk factors alone. This chapter concentrates

---

N. Ahmad (✉)
Manchester University Foundation Trust, Manchester, UK

Translational Medicine, University of Manchester, Manchester, UK

Greater Manchester and East Cheshire Strategic Clinical Network, Manchester, UK
e-mail: Naseer.Ahmad@mft.nhs.uk

F. Lee Bowling
Manchester University Foundation Trust, Manchester, UK

Translational Medicine, University of Manchester, Manchester, UK

World Health Organisation, Diabetes Task Force Lead, Geneva, Switzerland

R. Mani
Academic Division of Human Health and Development, Faculty of Medicine, University of Southampton, Southampton, UK

Faculty of Medicine, Chiang Mai University, Chiang Mai, Thailand

Shanghai Jiao Tong University School of Medicine, Shanghai, China

R. Mani et al. (eds.), *Compression and Chronic Wound Management*,
https://doi.org/10.1007/978-3-030-01195-6_1

on the impact and treatment of wounds not on the individual but rather the population as a whole. In it the issue of limb amputation is considered as an example. Amputation is a common occurrence in patients with the diabetic foot. The chapter describes the principles that underpin public health research, particularly the importance of inequalities, and, the social determinants of health, to provide a comprehensive view on the burden of chronic wounds to the health economy of England. It finally suggests a 'whole systems' population-based solution to reduce this burden and relates all this to compression which is a mainstay of treatment for another common chronic wound, the venous leg ulcer.

1.1 What Principles Underpin Public Health and Its Research?

The role of public health is to improve the nation's health and well-being and to reduce inequalities [1]. It works at a population and organisation level to make people healthier and to reduce differences in outcomes by promoting healthier lifestyles, advising government and supporting action by local government, the National Health Service (NHS) and the public [1].

The principle underpinning public health research is enshrined by the World Health Organisation statement;

> *'the highest standards of health should be within reach of all, without distinction of race, religion, political belief, economic or social condition'*
>
> —World Health Organisation, 1946 [2]

There are many variations in health that are seen across populations and accepted such as older people being generally sicker than the young. However, other variations such as poorer outcomes in socially deprived children are seen but deemed unacceptable. Such variability is considered irreparable i.e. not within the immediate gift of individuals: this concept is defeatist and unacceptable. Health inequality occurs when such variations are systematic, socially produced and unfair [2].

The core concept underpinning health inequality research, therefore, is to understand and remove systemic unfairness within the system and to promote social justice. However, the term 'health inequality' itself is used to describe examples of both acceptable and unacceptable variations. Other inter-changeable terms commonly used are variation, disparity and inequity. Although, all these terms essentially describe difference, they do not imply injustice. Clarification is therefore required when using such terms. In this chapter, the term inequality, when used, is simply to describe difference and not imply systematic injustice.

The issue of inequality is significant within the NHS as healthcare in the UK is free at the point of delivery. There should, therefore, be parity in outcomes among disparate groups because there is no economic barrier to seeking and receiving treatment. However, a 'health gap' i.e. difference in health between the least and most deprived populations does exist in England and is significant [3].

1.2 The Health Gap Across England

The Office National Statistics (ONS) measured the health gap across England based on occupation from the 2011 census [3]. Social class was split into seven where class 1 were higher managerial and professional workers e.g. doctors, lawyers and architects and class 7 were workers such as labourers and bar staff. By comparing the health measure 'not good' between classes 1 and 7, the 'health gap' was calculated. Overall, the percentage of men reporting health as 'not good' was 13.7 in class 1 and 30.5 in class 7- the difference of 16.8 is the health gap. Figure 1.1 describes the health gap by region in men and women. It shows greater health inequality in the North compared with Southern England and in women compared with men [3].

Health inequality also places a major financial burden on government spending. The Marmot report reviewed the cost of health inequality in illness and reported that it costs the British economy around £32bn each year in productivity losses, £25bn in lost taxes and welfare payments, and £5.5bn in additional health care costs [4]. The cause of these inequalities is multi-factorial. It includes the traditional biological modifiable and non-modifiable causes, but, additionally, and with increasing awareness, includes the social determinants of health.

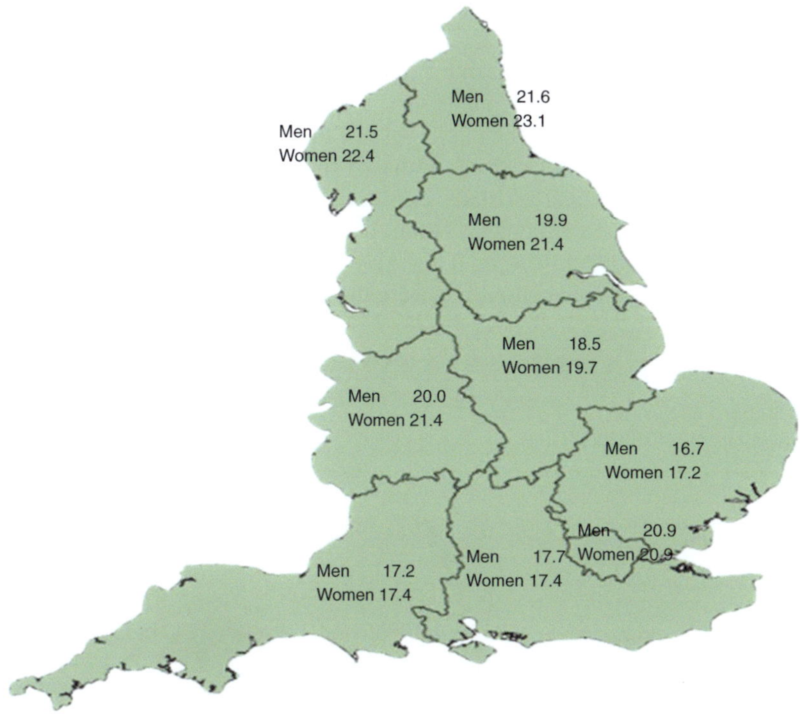

Fig. 1.1 Health Gap between the least and most deprived populations across England; Men and Women based on census 2011 [3]

1.3 The Social Determinants of Health

The 'social determinants of health' model [2] (Fig. 1.2) describes the multi-factorial cause of ill health and links the biological and social causes. The model itself is a multi-layer framework with the individual at the centre surrounded by health modifying factors of reducing personal control.

The model acknowledges the responsibility of the individual but incorporates the roles of health professionals and government in creating an environment where health is promoted. Policies that seek to improve health outcomes, therefore, need to address these social determinants in addition to the biological, lifestyle and treatment factors.

Health professionals traditionally view their role as influencing individuals by encouraging them to take up healthier lifestyles thus addressing modifiable risk factors. However, professionals can also influence the system and ensure health care services have parity in both provision and quality. The whole systems analysis discussed later aims to bring together all these determinants of health.

1.3.1 The Burden of Chronic Wounds in England

Chronic wounds are an increasing burden on the health system. The diagnosis and economic cost of 135,000 wounds seen across 513 General Practices was investigated by Guest et al. and then extrapolated to the general population of England [5]. They defined a chronic wound based on its diagnosis rather than duration which is often difficult to state with accuracy. Overall 60% of wounds were chronic with the main diagnosis being 'ulcers' which were of 'venous', 'diabetic foot' and 'pressure' in origin. They also included 'acute' wounds which were categorised based on whether they were the result of an abscess, trauma, burns or

Fig. 1.2 The Social Determinants of Health [2]

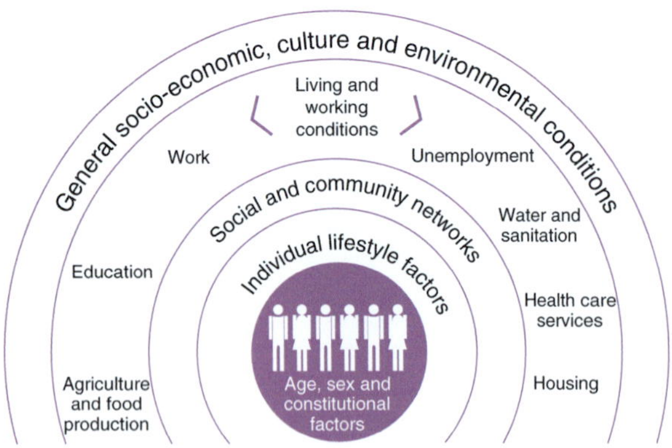

Table 1.1 Classification of chronic wounds in general practice [5]

Type of wounds	Percentage of all wounds (%)
Leg ulcer (unspecified)	19
Leg ulcer (venous)	13
Diabetic foot ulcer	8
Pressure Ulcer	7
Unspecified	12
Acute e.g. abscess, burns, trauma	41

Table 1.2 Distribution of costs (percentage of total) for the management of acute, chronic and unspecified wounds [6]

	Type of Wound			
	Acute[a] (%)	Chronic[b] (%)	Unspecified (%)	All wounds (%)
Community costs				
Community nurse visits	8	15	16	13
GP visits	6	7	8	7
Practice Nurse visits	4	5	5	5
Specialist nurse visits	<1	<1	0	<1
Allied Health Care visits	<1	1	2	1
Hospital costs				
Hospital admission and day cases	42	11	14	23
Hospital outpatients	7	7	13	8
Investigations and products				
Drug Prescriptions	14	28	25	23
Wound care products	12	15	12	14
Devices	3	6	2	5
Diagnostic tests	2	4	5	3
Other	<1	<1	<1	<1

[a]Burns/Abscess/Trauma or wounds that take >4 weeks to heal post-surgery
[b]Diabetes foot and leg ulcers

surgically induced but taking longer than 4 weeks to heal. Table 1.1 provides a detailed breakdown of these wounds.

The economic costs of these wounds and patient co-morbidities, extrapolated to the population of England, at 2013/2014 prices, was approximately £6bn [6]. The costs were split into those originating in the community and those when patients were admitted into hospital. The main costs were drug prescriptions, community nurse visits and hospital visits (Table 1.2) [6].

Guest et al. determined also that over the course of a year, only 43% of chronic wounds healed and that prevalence was rising at approximately 12% per year [6]. These figures and the corresponding burden of wounds was debated in the House of Lords in November 2017 where it was concluded that the burden of wounds on the NHS was greater than that of obesity and that a national strategy was required [7].

1.4 What is the Inequality in Outcome Surrounding Chronic Wounds

There are no national data describing the inequality in outcome surrounding wound care management. However, as the majority of amputations in those aged 50 and over are due to chronic wounds (5% are related to trauma and cancer [8]), the variation in lower limb amputation rates may serve as a proxy measure.

The prevalence of major amputation in England, among those aged 50–84, is, approximately 26/100,000 [9]. however rates across England vary by 50% with prevalence higher in Northern England compared with the South (Fig. 1.3) [9]. In addition to this, the above to below knee amputation ratio is also higher in Northern regions (North 1.3:1, Midlands 1.2:1, South 0.9:1) [10]. This North/South divide mirrors the heath gap. However, in addition to this divide, the amputation rate is nearly three higher in men than women and 70% higher in the Black population [11]. The reasons for this variation is unknown, however, the prevalence of co-morbidities such as diabetes and peripheral arterial disease, the main causes of these ulcers, do not show such variation [12, 13]. It is interesting to note that the prevalence of major lower limb amputation in South Asians i.e. those of Indian, Pakistani, Bangladeshi or Sri Lankan origin is 40% lower than the 'White' and 'Black' populations of England despite much higher levels of diabetes [11].

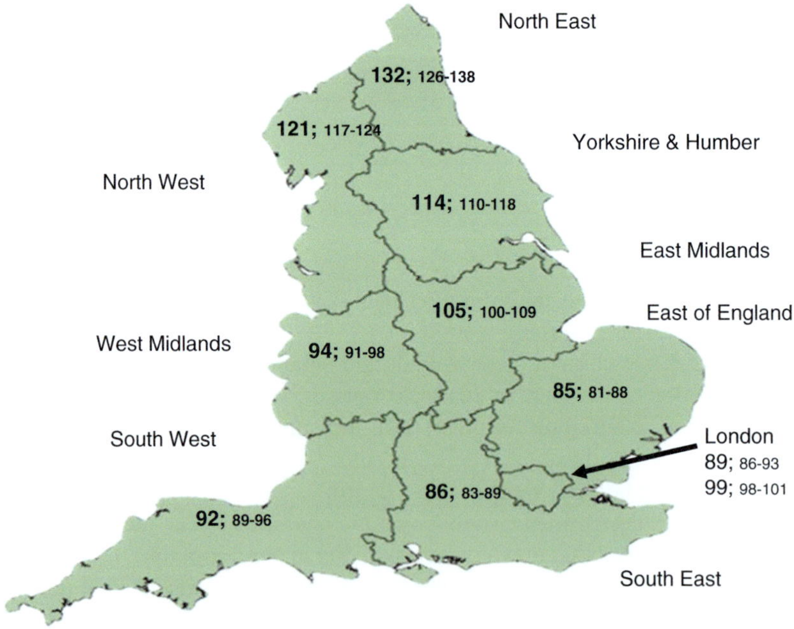

Fig. 1.3 Proportional percentage prevalence (relative to national average; England = 100) of lower limb major amputation; Males and Females aged 50–84: England 2003–2009 [9]

One reason for the variation, the correction of which lies within the gift of health professionals is the way in which conditions are treated. Disparate systems of treatment even within close geographical areas exist and harmonising services to reduce inequity in provision is a starting point to reducing inequalities in outcome.

1.5 Principles Behind a 'Whole Systems Approach' to Improving Wound Care

One of the main barriers to harmonising services is that competing NHS areas (often contiguous), have very different priorities and budgets. This is not conducive to cross border co-operation within the larger NHS 'family'. A 'whole systems analysis' is a relatively new concept in healthcare which aims to overcome this hurdle. This term as well as the resulting 'whole systems flow' is used to define the coordination of all processes, systems and resources across an entire local health and social care economy, to deliver effective, efficient, person-centred care in the right setting at the right time and by the right person [14]. The term 'health and social care economy' refers to those organisations e.g. hospitals, community clinics, social care services etc. that provide services across a defined geographical area. Improving the flow of patients, information and resources within and between health and social care organisations has a crucial role to play in driving up service quality and productivity [14].

1.6 A Potential 'Whole Systems Flow Model' Applied to Wound Care: The Manchester Amputation Reduction Strategy (MARS Project)

The concept of whole systems analysis, as applied to wound care, is being developed in Greater Manchester. This region has a population of 2.8 million spread across ten clinical commissioning groups and has some of the most deprived areas in the country. Approximately 1000 major and minor amputations are performed annually with the national inequalities also seen regionally. The major amputation rate is 36% above the national average and to address this 'The Manchester Amputation Reduction Strategy (The MARS Project) is currently being developed. This aims to reduce amputations through coordinated high quality care of foot and leg ulcers. It additionally aims to reduce inequity in service provision and cost whilst improving patient flow and incorporate Public Health and Social Care [15].

The economic cost of wound care based on the costings by Guest et al. [6] applied to the population of Greater Manchester [16] and extrapolated forward using NHS Inflation figures [17] is shown in Table 1.3. It shows the cost to be £213m

Table 1.3 Rising cost of wound care in Greater Manchester area 2017/18 to 2021/22 [6, 16, 17]

	Estimated Cost of Wound Care over 5 years[a]		
Type of Wound	2017/2018	2019/2020	2021/2022
Chronic Wounds[b] (excl. comorbidities)	213,624,897	271,913,221	356,225,512
Chronic Wounds (incl. comorbidities)[c]	273,648,841	346,614,270	456,905,751
Acute and Chronic[d] (incl. comorbidities)	357,536,830	449,694,444	579,249,247

[a]Based on applying data from Guest et al. [6] and incorporating projected annual health inflation as per NHS Improvement [16]

[b]Defined by diagnosis not duration and includes foot/leg ulcers and 'unspecified' as per Table 1.1 (excludes acute wounds)

[c]Cost of managing co-morbidities of patients with chronic wounds

[d]Cost of managing all wounds (acute, chronic and unspecified) and associated comorbidities of patients

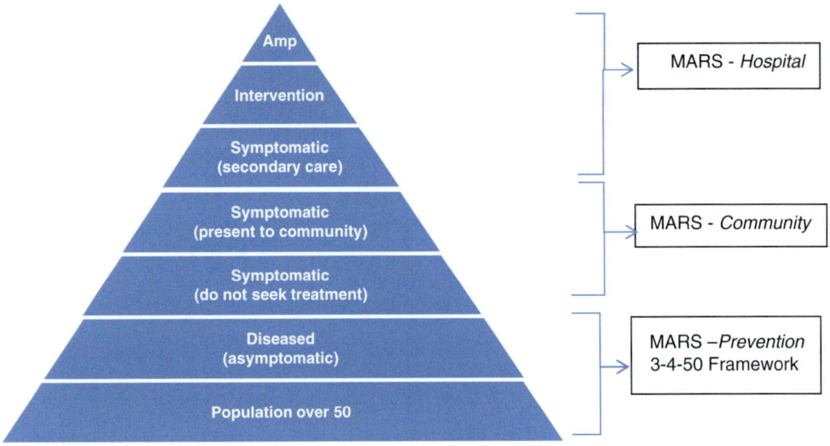

Fig. 1.4 Iceberg of disease burden leading to an amputation and the Whole Systems MARS solution

in 2017/2018 and is expected to rise to £356m by 2021/22. The management of these patients' co-morbidities will require an additional £100m by 2021/22. These figures show the importance of reducing not only the prevalence of chronic wounds but preventing the co-morbidities that give rise to these ulcers.

The MARS plan acknowledges that an amputation is the culmination of a number of steps. Therefore each phase requires an intervention (Fig. 1.4).

Amputations represent the tip of the iceberg of disease and reducing amputation requires a collaborative Public Health, Community, Hospital and Social care. Mental Health services are also aligned in the community hub of this model. The aim of the 'community arm' of the MARS model is to reduce the heterogeneity of service provision surrounding community foot and leg ulcer management. The current multiple referral pathways are summarised in Fig. 1.5. A proposed harmonised MARS pathway is shown in Fig. 1.6.

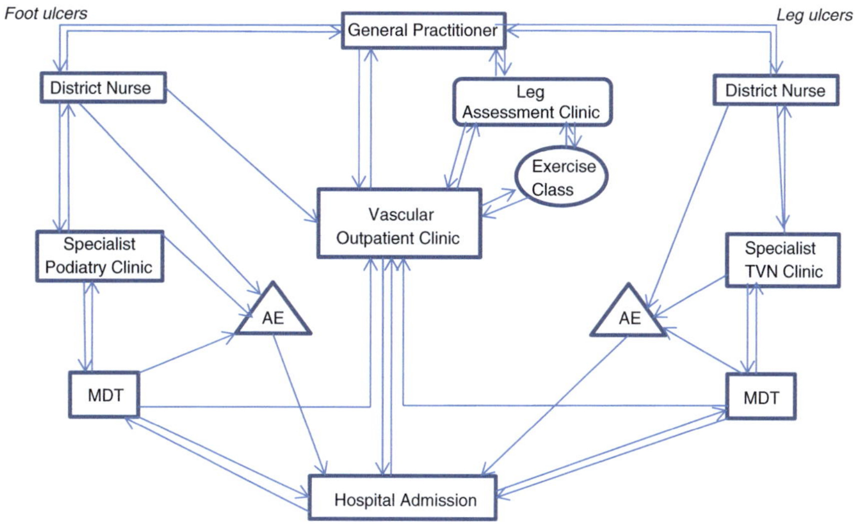

Fig. 1.5 The Current Foot and Leg Service

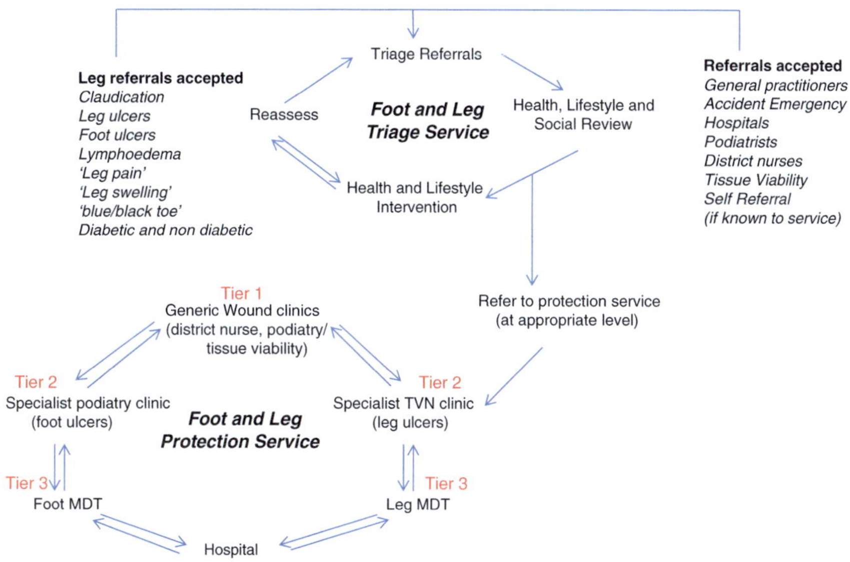

Fig. 1.6 The Proposed MARS Foot and Leg Service

Here, there are two components; a 'Triage Service' and a 'Protection Service'. The Triage Service will triage, diagnose, and treat the population at risk. It will undertake also the public health, social and mental health care needs assessment. In line with the MARS Public Health Framework the triage service will offer lifestyle and risk factor modification programs and be the centre for health promotion in the community for this high risk population. Patients with foot and leg ulcers will be referred to the Protection Service. Here, there will be three tiers of management; tier 1 (District Nurse level) will manage the most basic of wounds, tier 2 (Specialist clinics) will be run by Specialist Podiatrists and Tissue Viability Nurses with the most complex wounds managed at the multi-disciplinary level (tier 3). Tier 1 and 2 will be in the community and tier 3 in hospital outpatient setting. Patients will move through the tiers seamlessly as the wounds progress or regress. The three tiers will be part of one wound care team with healthcare professionals rotating through all tiers in order to support, spread confidence and improve equality in management. It is envisioned that the community wound care teams will be managed by Non Medical Consultants and be integrated with hospital teams.

1.7 How Does This Relate to Compression and Chronic Wounds?

Chronic wound management relies on the delivery of standardised care and this is based on a reliable diagnosis and treatment of the underlying cause and a new model for care is presented in Fig. 1.6. For venous leg ulcers, such treatment is based on limb compression delivered using elasticated bandages, garments or, as is now becoming clear, devices that promote venous return. The physics of compression as well as its use are dealt with extensively in other chapters in this book which also devotes chapters to devices that can provide compression by promoting venous return.

When standardised care fails to deliver an adequate rate of healing, the advice is to revisit the diagnosis, manage any complications and then return to the mainstay of management. Adjunct devices to promote wound healing are produced rapidly by innovators: the applicability of adjunct devices is best tested within the realms of standardised care [18]. Figures 1.5 and 1.6 describe pathways to achieve these steps. The MARS project although aimed at reducing amputations is actually about managing chronic wounds e.g. leg ulcers in a standard and high quality consistent way.

1.8 Summary

The prevalence and cost of chronic wounds is both significant and rising. As such, they represent a significant burden on individuals and society. Whilst improvements in treatment are crucial to better outcomes for individuals, a 'whole systems approach' is required to reduce inequality in outcome and ensuring all people get access to be best services. The MARS Project adopts such an approach and the results of this innovative cross sectoral collaborative approach to ulcer care eagerly awaited.

References

1. Public Health England. https://www.gov.uk/government/organisations/public-health-england/about. Last accessed 8 June 2018.
2. Whitehead M, Dahlgren G. Concepts and principles for tackling social inequities in health: Levelling up Part 1. World Health Organisation 2007. Available at http://www.euro.who.int/__data/assets/pdf_file/0010/74737/E89383.pdf. Last accessed 8 June 2018.
3. Office National Statistics. Health gap in England and Wales, 2011 Census. 2013. Available at http://www.ons.gov.uk/ons/rel/census/2011-census-analysis/health-gaps-by-socio-economic-position-of-occupations-in-england%2D%2Dwales%2D%2Denglish-regions-and-local-authorities%2D%2D2011/info-health-gap.html. Last accessed 8 June 2018.
4. Marmot M. Fair Society Health Lives. HMSO 2010. Available at http://www.instituteofhealthequity.org/projects/fair-society-healthy-lives-the-marmot-review. Last accessed 8 June 2018.
5. Guest JF, Ayoub N, McIlwraith T, Uchegbu I, Garrish A, Weidlich D, Vowden K, Vowden P. Health economic burden that wounds impose on the national health service. BMJ Open. 2015;5:e009283. Last accessed 8 June 2018.
6. Guest JF, Vowden K, Vowden P. The health economic burden that acute and chronic wounds impose on an average clinical commissioning group/health board in the UK. J Wound Care. 2017;26:292–303.
7. Hansard. Debate in House of Lords 22 November 2017. Available at https://hansard.parliament.uk/Lords/2017-11-22/debates/6C57E65A-A04D-449B-82E9-C836F088A696/NHSWoundCare. Last accessed 8 June 2018.
8. The Amputee Statistical Database for the United Kingdom 2006/2007. Information Service Division NHS Scotland Edinburgh 2009. www.limbless-statistics.org/documents/Report2006-07.pdf. Last accessed 8 June 2018.
9. Ahmad N, Thomas GN, Gill P, Chan C, Torella F. Lower limb amputation in England: prevalence, regional variation and relationship with revascularisation, deprivation and risk factors. A retrospective review of English hospital data. J R Soc Med. 2014;107(12):483–9.
10. Ahmad N, Thomas GN, Gill P, Torella F. Endovascular revascularisation is associated with a lower risk of above knee amputation than surgical or combined modalities. Analysis of English hospital admissions over a six year period. Int J Angiol. 2016;35:498–503.
11. Ahmad N, Chan C, Thomas GN, Gill P. Ethnic differences in lower limb revascularisation and amputation rates. Implications for the aetiopathology of atherosclerosis? Atherosclerosis. 2014;233:503–7.
12. Fowkes FGR, Rudan D, Rudan I, Aboyans V, Denenberg JO, McDermott MM, et al. Comparison of global estimates of prevalence and risk factors for peripheral artery disease in 2000 and 2010: a systematic review and analysis. Lancet. 2013;382:1329–40.
13. Health and Social Care Information Centre. Health and Lifestyle Survey 2014. Available at www.hscic.gov.uk/healthsurveyengland. Last accessed 8 June 2018.
14. Fillingham D, Jones B, Pereira P. The Challenge and potential of whole system flow. Improving the flow of people, information and resources across whole health and social care economies. The Health Foundation 2016. Available at https://www.health.org.uk/sites/health/files/ChallengeAndPotentialOfWholeSystemFlow.pdf. Last accessed 8 June 2018.
15. Ahmad N. Introducing the Manchester Amputation Reduction Strategy. The need for a cross sectoral, collaborative, whole systems analysis of services that leads to saving legs. Podiatry Now. 2017;7:28–31.
16. Office National Statistics. Clinical Commissioning Group mid year population estimates 2016. Available at https://www.ons.gov.uk/peoplepopulationandcommunity/populationandmigration/populationestimates/datasets/clinicalcommissioninggroupmidyearpopulationestimates. Last accessed 8 June 2018.
17. NHS Improvement. Economic assumptions 2016/17 to 2020/21. Available at https://improvement.nhs.uk/resources/economic-assumptions-1617-to-2021/. Last accessed 8 June 2018.
18. Mani R, Margolis DJ, Shukla VK, et al. Optimising the use of technology to manage chronic lower extremity wounds: a consensus document. Int J Low Extrem Wounds. 2015;15(2):102–19.

Chapter 2
Physics of Using Compression to Treat Venous Leg Ulcers and Other Conditions of the Lower Extremities

Hugo Partsch and Raj Mani

Abstract Compression is the mainstay of management of ambulatory venous hypertension, the most common sequel of which is venous leg ulceration. The logic for selecting compression is based on physical principles governing tension, pressure, volume as elegantly enshrined in the works of French mathematician philosophers Laplace and prior to him, Pascal. The application of Laplace's law for using compression bandages to manage limb swelling consequent to unrelieved venous pressures and sequelae are described and used with Pascal's law to comprehend the limitations of compression systems. While robust data from several reports endorse the concept of using compression, evidence also indicates the limitations of and difficulties encountered in practice of offering compression which involve, to a large part, changing position: from lying still to standing upright and being ambulant. The concept of measuring static stiffness index (SSI), described by Partsch, helps to explain these changes. SSI should be measured with the patient upstanding and at a specific point on the calf. This and guidance for offering compression for other clinical conditions are described in this chapter.

Keywords Compression · Tension · Pressure · Static stiffness index · Venous leg ulcers · Bandaging systems

---

H. Partsch (✉)
Emeritus Professor, Medical University of Vienna, Vienna, Austria
e-mail: Hugo.Partsch@meduniwien.ac.at

R. Mani
Academic Division of Human Health and Development, Faculty of Medicine, University of Southampton, Southampton, UK

Faculty of Medicine, Chiang Mai University, Chiang Mai, Thailand

Shanghai Jiao Tong University School of Medicine, Shanghai, China
e-mail: rm1@soton.ac.uk

R. Mani et al. (eds.), *Compression and Chronic Wound Management*,
https://doi.org/10.1007/978-3-030-01195-6_2

2.1 Introduction

Compression is essential to treat venous hypertension and its sequalae. A great proportion of our current knowledge is derived from the use of bandages and garments to deliver compression to limbs. In order to fully comprehend the delivery and effects of such compression, it is important to define certain basic concepts of physics applicable to limb compression.

The laws of compression as defined by Laplace (1749–1827) a French Scholar (whose mathematical explanations of forces contributed to mechanics) as well Pascal's (seventeenth century French Mathematician and Scholar) equations relating to transmission of forces, are central to this understanding.

The use of externally applied compression to human limbs, in this book the focus is on lower legs, is to counteract excess pressures that develop within consequent to damage or dysfunction within venous valves, or congenital changes. The excess pressure that results from such dysfunction is often exacerbated when the calf muscle pump fails thereby losing an in-built pressure relieving mechanism. Changes to skin and tissue that follow leading to cell death and ulceration are well described in the literature and other chapters in this book. Routine management of this condition is contingent on externally delivering pressure is achieved using bandages. To better understand the use of such a common treatment effect, the relevant essentials of physics are first explained in this chapter.

2.1.1 *Definitions*

Through the lens of mechanics, **compression (or squeezing)** is the application of balanced inward forces to different points on a material or structure.

Pressure is defined by the Force applied perpendicularly to the surface of an object per unit area over which that force is distributed. In the medical field, pressure is expressed mainly mmHg, a common example is blood pressure. Formerly and in some societies, pressure was expressed in Pascals the conversion multiplier being (1 mmHg = 133.3 Pa, 1 Pa = 1 N = 1 kg/m^2).

2.1.2 *Laplace's Law*

When a bandage is wrapped around a human limb (leg or arm), the inward pushing force or the compression pressure P is dependent on the amount of bandage stretch as well as the *curvature* of the limb. The amount of bandage 'stretch', or Tension, which is transmitted tangentially to the limb depends on the elastic properties of the material of which the bandage or garment is made [1, 2]. As human limbs may be approximated to be cylindrical in cross section, it is reasonable to use limb radius, R, as a measure of its circumference which is especially important when considering compressing limbs.

The compression pressure P applied is *directly* proportional to the tension in bandage (*T*) and *inversely* proportional to the radius of the curvature of the limb under compression. In physics this approximation may be presented as $P = KT/R$ where K is an experimental constant, T is the bandage tension and R the limb radius. According to the law of Laplace, compression pressure will be zero over completely flat areas (since Radius of a flat surface is infinity), while it will be high over sharp edges (since Radius is tending to zero as the surface shape tends to sharp edges) (Fig. 2.1).

The pressure perceived beneath a bandage is also governed by its width as well as number of layers applied: the pressure of each layer of bandage of the same width will add to the total pressure on skin beneath. The law of Laplace has important applications:

- When bandaging a skinny lower leg, caution must be exercised not to excessively stretch the compressive material as this would increase the pressure P perceived on skin: contrariwise, in swollen legs with a higher radius, the bandage should be applied with much higher tension (T) to achieve a comparable pressure P. In other words, the same bandage when applied with the same tension will exert greater tension over a skinny leg than a swollen one. Be careful while wrapping bandages over a skinny leg. Note, it is equally important to be careful while wrapping bandages around a swollen limb for fear of damaging the skin.

If the tension in the compression garment is the same throughout, the applied pressure will decrease with increasing circumference. A good way to remember this is the example of stringing the handle of a cricket bat which is uniformly cylindrical. It must be wrapped around tightly using twine held as tightly as possible (ten-

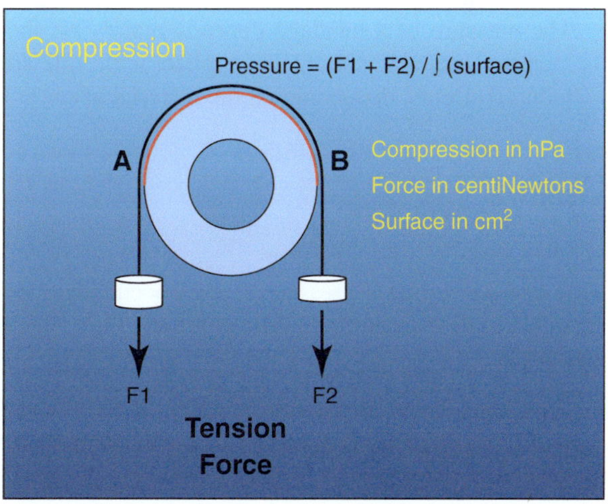

Fig. 2.1 Diagrammatic representation of Laplace's law. P = PRESSURE; usually given in mmHg or in Pascal T = tension, force in Newton per unit width. R = Radius of the limb segment (cm). (1 Pa = 1 N/m^2 = 10.000 N/s cm^2 = 7.35 mmHg/cm^2)

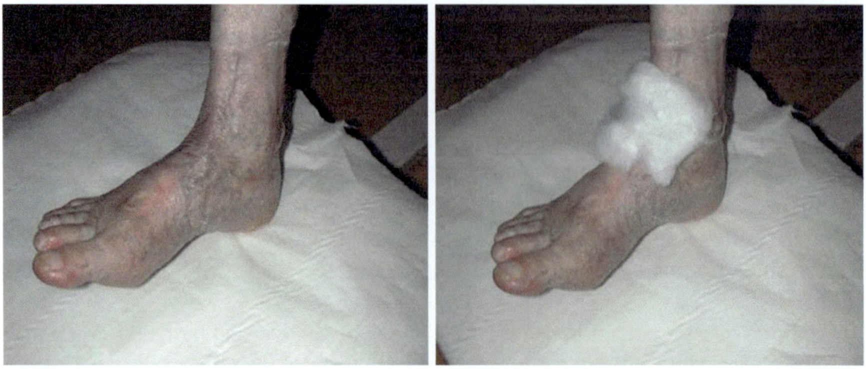

Fig. 2.2 Padding the tendon by cotton wool is recommended to decrease the local compression pressure (by increasing the radius of the leg segment)

sion is kept constant and high) while the bat is rotated slowly leaving a layer or more of equally tensioned, equally spaced string that is comfortable to grip.

Returning to bandaging human limbs, increasing or decreasing the radii of surfaces bandaged offers protective effects, a good application of Laplace's Law.

- To protect the tendon elevating the foot, bandages should be applied during maximal dorsiflexion and the protruding tendon should be padded by applying some cotton wool to enlarge the site radius (= reduce local pressure as figuratively shown in Fig. 2.2).
- To increase local pressure over flat parts of the extremity the local curvature can be made smaller by using pads ("eccentric compression") thereby increasing the local pressure over a hematoma or a painful phlebitis reaction after sclerotherapy or endovenous procedure. The same may be advisable to increase the local pressure over a retro- malleolar ulcer where locally applied pads will increase the pressure. Figures 2.8 and 2.9 shows a clinical example where local pads (not shown) led to healing.
- The pressure of a bandage depends mainly on the stretch during application: inelastic material should be applied with full stretch, elastic material with reduced stretch, depending on the material used.

2.1.3 Pascals Law

This law states that a pressure change occurring anywhere in a confined incompressible fluid is transmitted throughout the fluid such that the same change occurs everywhere.

- Using inelastic compression material, the sub- bandage pressure will increase with every increase of the extremity volume due to muscle contraction. This will lead to massaging effects during walking. Changes in limb circumference have an immediate effect on the amount of pressure provided.

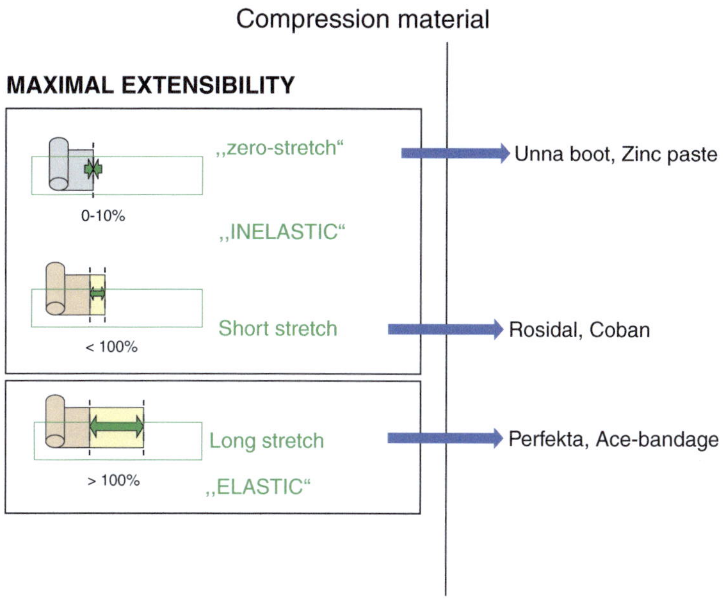

Fig. 2.3 Schematic classification of compression material depending on the maximal extensibility, examples on the right side

2.2 Compression Materials

In principle three types of compression material can be differentiated [3]:

No stretch (maximal extensibility 0–5%)
Short stretch (maximal extensibility <100%)
Long stretch I (Maximal extensibility >100%)

Figure 2.3 shows some examples.

2.2.1 Pressure

When using compression stockings, we are reliant on the pressure range data provided by manufacturers. Such pressure ranges are related to leg size. Different classes of compression exist and are based on in vitro measurements performed using extensometers [4]. We have suggested that compression garments be classified in mmHg since the classification of compression classes varies among countries at least in international publications [4] (see Table 2.1).

Applying compression bandages the exerted pressure depends on the stretch during application and not on the material.

Table 2.1 Compression pressure ranges (mmHg) given in different national regulations

Compression Class	EU (CEN)	USA	UK (BS 6612)	France	Germany
A	10–14 (light)				
I	15–21 (mild)	15–20 (moderate)	14–17 (light)	10–15	18–21 (light)
II	23–32 (moderate)	20–30 (firm)	18–24 (medium)	15–20	23–32 (medium)
III	34–46 (strong)	30–40 (extra firm)	25–35 (strong)	20–36	34–46 (strong)
IV	>49 (very strong)	40+		>36	>49 (very strong)

More important for the individual patient is the actual pressure corresponding to the dosage of compression on the leg which nowadays can be measured by various instruments [5, 6]. Measuring compression pressure is recommended only for scientific reasons in studies and for training purposes, but not for routine.

In a consensus paper the so called B1 point was recommended as a preferred location on the leg to differentiate the properties of several compression materials on the individual patient [7]. This is the site where the medial gastrocnemius muscle turns into the tendinous part (12–15 cm above the medial malleolus.). At this site, the circumference of the leg may be approximated as circular so that a point measurement of the pressure may be representative for the whole segment. In addition, this is the point on the lower leg which reflects the most extensive changes of circumference of the leg during movement [8]. During dorsiflexion or when a patient stands, the tendon of the medial gastrocnemius muscle protrudes, which leads to a decrease of the local leg curvature and therefore to an increase of the local interface pressure as explained by Laplace's law.

2.2.2 *Stiffness*

Stiffness involves pressure change with respect to a change in limb size: it may be defined as the change (increase/decrease) in sub-bandage pressure per centimeter increase/decrease in the circumference of the leg [9]. This parameter characterizes the elastic property of a compression device; it also defines the relationship between resting and working pressures. When the calf muscle contracts, an inelastic material will produce a higher increase of interface pressure than elastic or yielding material.

Static Stiffness Index is the difference between standing pressure and the pressure in the supine position exerted by compression material measured at the B1 point [10]. This difference will be low (up to 5 mmHg) for yielding, elastic material, for example a compression stocking, but high for inelastic bandages (e.g. 30 mmHg under a zinc paste bandage).

Thus, interface pressure is not constant, rather it varies with position and therefore with walking.

Table 2.2 Low and high stiffness compression materials

Low stiffness	High stiffness
Compression stockings	Rigid bandages (e.g. zinc paste), Velcro-band devices, pumps
Single component elastic bandages	Short stretch bandages, adhesive, cohesive material
	Multi-component bandages

To achieve the same pressure peaks during walking, elastic material would need to be applied with a much higher pressure which would not be tolerated in the resting position. Stiffness may be measured in the laboratory where it corresponds to the slope of the hysteresis curve. The fact that it can also be assessed by in-vivo measurements on the individual leg is of increasing practical importance [5] (Table 2.2).

As shown in Fig. 2.4 inelastic material produces a much higher pressure increase on standing up than elastic material. When several layers of elastic material are applied over each other stiffness of the final bandage will increase. This is also true for elastic stockings applied over each other [5]. Adhesive and cohesive materials increase stiffness.

2.2.3 Graduation of Pressure Along a Limb

The concept of a graduated or 'degressive' pressure assumes that under physiological conditions venous flow occurs from distally to proximally or from high pressure to a lower pressure: thus, creating a reverse pressure gradient by applying higher proximal compression would impede venous return [11]. While this concept holds good for a lower limb at rest, it may be questioned for the mobile patient: during walking when the calf muscles contract, intramuscular pressures may rise to 200–250 mmHg [12, 13]. Higher pressures over the calf compared to distal parts of the leg have been reported to increase the ejection fraction of the calf pump more in patients with chronic venous insufficiency compared to those using graduated compression [14, 15].

Wearing "anti-gradient stockings" some swelling of the foot may occur after bed rest but will this will disappear when the patient starts walking.

2.2.4 Application and Maintenance

Compression stockings are mainly indicated to prevent and/or reduce leg swelling, while stockings or garments made from inelastic material applied with higher pressure are preferable to improve the venous hemodynamics in patients with venous incompetence, but also to decongest lymphedema limbs in the initial treatment phase.

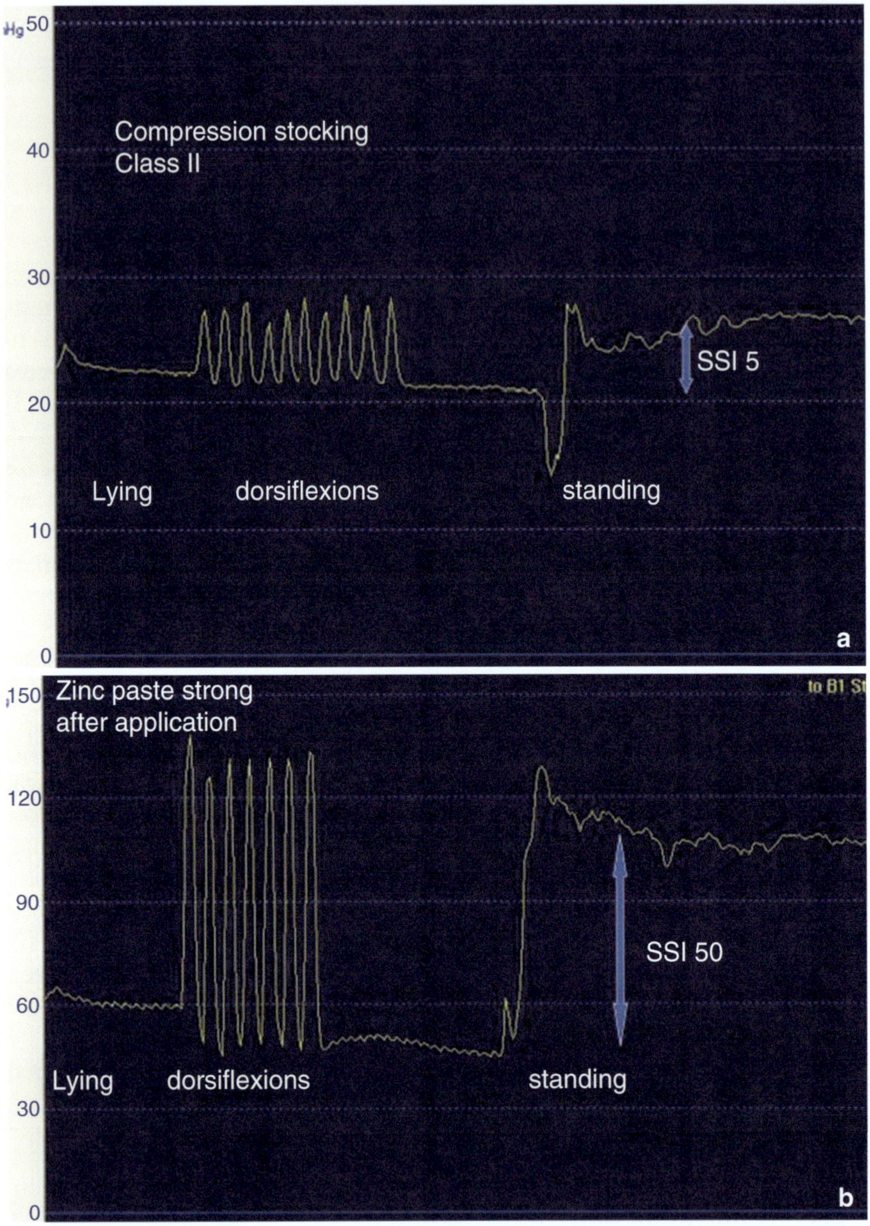

Fig. 2.4 (**a**) Compression pressure measured under a compression stocking at B1 level in the supine position, with dorsiflexions and after standing up. SSI = "Static stiffness index" is the difference between standing and lying pressure. (**b**) Compression pressure measured under a tightly applied zinc paste bandage: much higher amplitudes of pressure with dorsi flexions ("massaging effect") and after standing up resulting in much higher SSI may be observed

The proper donning and doffing of compression stockings may cause problems: which is frequently limiting patients' compliance with such therapeutic devices.

For elderly patients, pulling on or taking off compression stockings may well be difficult especially for those with restricted mobility and/or joint problems in the fingers, in the hip and spine which make bending down to the feet problematic. This consideration will apply for obese patients who find bending down to the reach their feet difficult due to increased girth. Stocking manufacturers offer several devices that are helpful [16]. Using several layers of light stockings over each other may help to achieve sufficient compression as the pressure exerted by each layer adds [17].

Stronger compression stockings are not tolerated in the lying position and therefore need to be removed before going to bed and to be reapplied in the morning. Usually this should be done by the patients themselves, but due to the restrictions mentioned additional help from relatives or by nursing staff is often needed.

Compression bandages need to be applied by specifically trained practitioners. A key cause of limited clinical effects of compression bandages is poor bandaging technique. The main point is the exerted stretch during application as well as the addition to the number of layers rather than mode of wrapping the bandage around which may be circular or in figure of eight fashion (Spica").

Inelastic bandages should be applied over a padding foam layer to prevent slippage.

Several studies have shown that most bandages are applied too loosely [18, 19]. It should be noted that bandage garment pressure will reduce as limb edema reduces and this is more obvious when bandages are made from stiff materials. Materials with hook and loop fasteners (Velcro-wraps) are effective alternatives to avoid these draw-backs: They can be applied with high pressure by the trained patient and re-adjusted when getting loose [20].

2.3 Effects of Compression

2.3.1 Compression Effects on Venous Circulation

The effect of compression on veins depends on the intravenous pressure which is variable, depending mainly on the body position. The hydrostatic pressure in a peripheral vein is the product of the vertical distance of the peripheral vein from the right atrium and the specific gravity of the blood. In an elevated extremity, veins will collapse, and the intravenous pressure will only be slightly higher than that of the surrounding tissues, while in a dependent position the pressure will correspond to the weight of the blood column between the measuring site and the right heart. In the standing position the pressure in a dorsal foot vein in a person with normal body height is between 80 and 100 mmHg, in the popliteal vein around 60 mmHg and in the femoral vein around 30 mmHg (Fig. 2.5) [21].

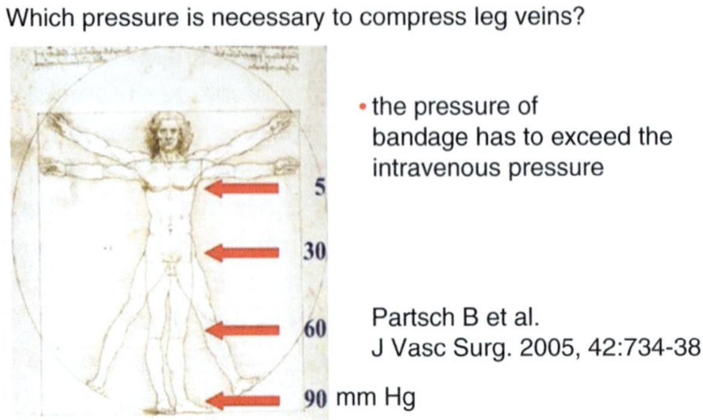

Fig. 2.5 Intravenous pressures measured at different levels in the standing position, corresponding to the weight of the blood column between the measuring point and the right heart

If we wish to compress a lower leg vein in the standing position the external pressure of a compression device should be higher than the local venous blood pressure, which is more than 60 mmHg [22, 46].

During movement the situation is getting much more complex. Muscle contractions lead to an increase in the muscle compartment pressure to more than 150 mmHg which will collapse the intramuscular veins. Depending on the competence of the vein valves there is a reduction of the peripheral venous pressure during walking due to the blood pumped up towards the heart. If the veins are incompetent there is an up and down movement of blood in the veins and their mean pressure will not fall. This constellation is called "ambulatory venous hypertension" which is the deciding key parameter characterizing the severity of chronic venous disease.

By measuring ambulatory venous hypertension in patients with severe CVI due to massive venous reflux it could be demonstrated that external -compression peaks of more than 70 mmHg are able to reduce this elevated intravenous pressure [23] (see Fig. 2.6). Since this could also be demonstrated in patients with congenital absence of vein valves this improvement cannot be explained by re-approaching defect valves, but rather by a hemodynamic effect creating a functional valve mechanism [24].

To achieve a high enough compression pressure during walking only elastic material applied with sufficient resting pressure (50 mmHg or more) will work. However, a standing pressure of 70 mmHg achieved by elastic material would not be tolerated by the patient during rest.

2.3.2 *Compression Effects on Arterial Circulation*

Measuring the arm blood pressure, we use a cuff which is blown up to supra-systolic values and interrupt the arterial inflow. From this basic experience it is obvious that the compression pressure should never exceed the arterial perfusion pressure as this might happen in patients with severe arterial occlusive disease. In those cases, the

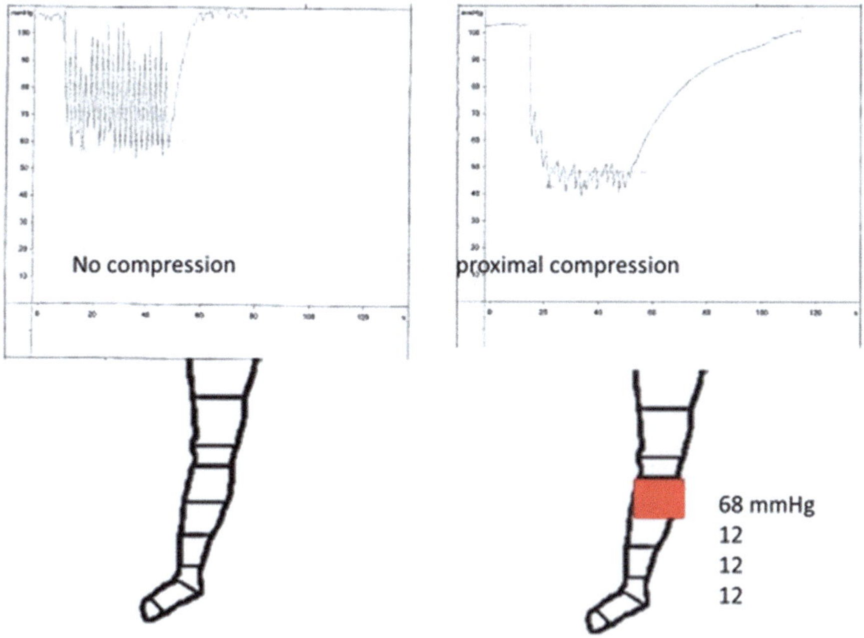

Fig. 2.6 Pressure measured in a dorsal foot vein in a patient with severe chronic venous insufficiency. Left: without compression during walking the pressure fall is severely restricted during muscle systole ("ambulatory venous hypertension"). After applying pressure to the calf (68 mmHg over the calf) the intravenous pressure is clearly more reduced during walking, especially during muscle systole and venous refilling is prolonged

systolic ankle pressure measured by a Doppler probe is a valuable indicator for the severity of the arterial occlusive disease. It is obvious that a compression pressure of 50 mmHg may block arterial inflow in cases with a systolic ankle pressure of the same amount, independent from the systolic arm pressure.

An increase of arterial flow under "mild" compression had been demonstrated not only in healthy people [25], but also, in vascular patients, questioning the dogma that compression will always reduce arterial inflow [26].

In patients with moderate arterial occlusions (systolic ankle pressure >50 mmHg, ABPI 0.6–0.80) compression applied with a pressure up to 40 mmHg has been shown to increase local blood flow and to promote the function of the calf muscle pumping in "mixed arterial-venous cases" with concomitant venous disease [27].

Specially constructed intermittent pressure pumps have shown amazing beneficial results not only in acute experiments but also in the long time run, demonstrating the development of new collaterals and increasing ankle pressure values after months [28, 29].

While the precise mechanisms governing these changes continue to be debated, there is no doubt the changes are perceived in the microcirculation of skin.

2.3.3 Compression Effects on Microcirculation

Increasing evidence shows that compression provides an "anti- inflammatory" effect. Slow flow in the venules due to venous hypertension is associated with a margination and increasing attachment of leucocytes to the endothelium which then will penetrate the vein wall and enter the surrounding tissue. Neutrophils release harmful mediators, including free radicals and proteases, which disrupt normal venous structure and function. It is likely that compression will impede neutrophil activation and attachment to the vein wall which in turn could have beneficial effects in reducing the inflammation. The most convincing experiments showing an improvement of the microcirculation were performed by using intermittent pneumatic pumps.

An intermittent acceleration of microcirculatory flow will increase the shear stress, which releases anti-inflammatory, vasodilating and antithrombotic substances from the endothelial cells [30].

This same effect also causes an increased shear stress on arterial endothelial cells when the sudden decrease in the venous pressure causes an increase in the A–V pressure gradient leading to an increased arterial flow velocity.

It may be assumed that the effects shown in these experiments are also relevant for the intermittent increase of pressure under inelastic compression material during movement (massaging effect).

Mani studied tissue hypoxia in venous conditions using skin surface sensors to measure transcutaneous oxygen tension ($TcPO_2$) at 43–44 °C and argued that tissue oxygen is dependent *directly* on oxygen delivered (in cutaneous perfusion) and *indirectly* on oxygen consumed (overcoming local infection) as well as resistance to the diffusion of oxygen in tissue [31]. Edema, a common complication in this condition will have the effect of increasing inter-capillary distances. Arguably therefore, reduction of edema will reduce distances between nutritional capillaries and tissue cells thereby improving the oxygen supply to the tissue [32, 33]. Barnes and Mani in a study of patients with chronic venous leg ulcers, demonstrated that passive leg elevation at 10^0 significantly reduced leg volumes and therefore leg circumference: these changes were associated with significant increases in peri-wound perfusion and oxygen diffusion. These findings lend support to the view that compression benefits local wound nutrition since it (compression) reduces leg edema and circumference [34]. Apelqvist argues that an increase in peri-wound $TcPO_2$ of 10 mmHg (from 20 to 30 mmHg) doubles the probability of wound healing without amputation. $TcPO_2$ levels above 40 mmHg are safe, below 20 mmHg are not consistent with tissue survival [35]. Apelqvist's data of non invasive evaluations were derived from skin around diabetic foot ulcers: the thresholds of $TcPO_2$ for use in chronic wound management do hold good [35] (Fig. 2.7).

Some studies showed an increase of transcutaneous oxygen tension ($TcPO_2$) after compression therapy [27, 33, 34, 36].

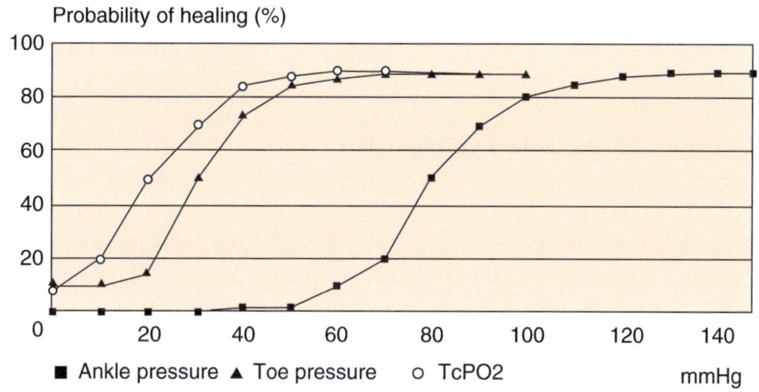

Fig. 2.7 This figure shows the relationships between systolic pressure (measured using Doppler ultrasound at the ankle) and skin perfusion pressure measured using Toe Pressure device and Transcutaneous oxygen tension and the probability of wound healing. Note the likelihood of healing increases significantly when skin perfusion pressure increases above 30 mmHg. It is also clear that Toe Pressures and Transcutaneous Oxygen tension measurements more sensitive to probability of wound healing

2.3.4 Compression Effects on Edema and Tissue Structure

Compression reduces capillary filtration and promotes the intrinsic contraction of lymph collectors.

2.3.4.1 Capillary Filtration

According to Starlings Law Capillary filtration depends on the balance between the hydrostatic pressure gradient and the oncotic pressure gradient across the capillary.

$$\text{Net Driving Pressure} = K\left[\left(P\text{c} - \text{Pi}\right) - \left(p\text{c} - p\text{i}\right)\right]$$

K = filtration coefficient, determined by the permeability of the vessel wall.

The four Starling's forces are:

- hydrostatic pressure in the capillary (Pc)
- hydrostatic pressure in the interstitium (Pi)
- oncotic pressure in the capillary (pc)
- oncotic pressure in the interstitium (pi)

The capillary hydrostatic pressure falls along the capillary from the arteriolar to the venous end and the driving pressure will decrease along the length of the capillary. The other Starling forces remain constant along the capillary.

The difference between the intra-venular pressure and the pressure from outside is the transmural pressure which will be reduced by external compression.

2.3.4.2 Contractions of the Lymphangion

Since lymphatics are regularly exposed to external forces and pulsations resulting in contraction/compression and relaxation cycles external pressure is a prerequisite for the normal functioning of the lymphatic drainage. While collapse of the initial lymphatics by external pressure is prevented by anchoring filaments or by elastic forces in the vessel wall unidirectional flow in lymphatics under normal conditions can only be observed during intrinsic contraction of a lymphatic and competent valves [37].

Oscillating forces transiently change the interstitial-intraluminal fluid pressure gradient, producing periodic movement into initial lymphatics. (It had been shown in a rabbit ear model that arterial pulsations were required for local lymphatic removal of subcutaneously injected tracer molecules, while steady perfusion of the artery at the same mean arterial pressure stopped lymph flow [38].

Also transient tissue deformation, due to activities such as walking, passive limb movements, or gentle skin massage promotes lymph clearance [37, 38].

The importance of oscillating forces explains why stiff compression material achieving a massaging effect due to muscular activity, but also with arterial pulsations is the preferred material in lymphedema patients.

Measuring compression pressure and intratympanic pressure in patients with lymphedema Olszewski found that raising cuff pressures caused increase of mean lymphatic pressure to 40–50 mmHg. There was no further increase in intralymphatic pressures even at external pressure of 80–100 mmHg. Contractions of calf muscles increased intralymphatic pressures to 110 mmHg at cuff pressure of 40 mmHg. Higher cuff pressures during calf muscle contractions did not have any additional effect on lymphatic pressure because the lymphangion's contracting force reached peak values [38].

2.3.4.3 Tissue Structure

In lymphedema there is progressive change of the skin texture as this becomes denser and harder. In course of time, fat is more and more replaced by fibrous tissue. Recurrent attacks of erysipelas lead to increase of post-inflammation collagen maturation and increased hardness of the skin.

Compression induces a change of the mechanical properties of the interstitium, mainly by shifting the liquid and gel compartments to non- compressed regions, where the fluid is moved towards normally functioning, valve-containing collecting vessels after entering the initial noncontractile lymphatics. It could be shown that skin texture measured by tissue dielectric constant and resistance assessed by tonometry can be improved by compression [39].

Zaleska and Olszewski showed that this fluid shift in severe stages of lymphedema happens mainly in spontaneously formed tissue channels showing no endothelial layers [40]. The bulk of edema fluid is located in the subcutis between stiff mature collagen bundles and fat globules can be reduced by IPC as demonstrated in studies using plethysmography [41, 42].

2.4 Compression Effects in Clinical Indications

2.4.1 Thromboprophylaxis (Anti-Stasis Action)

Based on the Triade of Virchow reduced blood flow velocity ("venous stasis) is one of the principle factors responsible for thrombosis (together with thrombophilic factors in the blood and endothelial damage). Compression leads to an increase of venous blood flow velocity which has been demonstrated by measuring the appearance time of injected isotopes and by Duplex investigations [43–45]. It could be shown that already very low external pressures exerted by so called thromboprophylactic stockings (TPS) are able to narrow veins in the lower extremity in the horizontal position (see Fig. 2.8) [6].

Narrowing of the great saphenous vein (in circle) and of the femoral vein (in square) can be seen.

However, the routine application of such stockings in bed ridden patients came into dispute after it has been demonstrated that in different indications

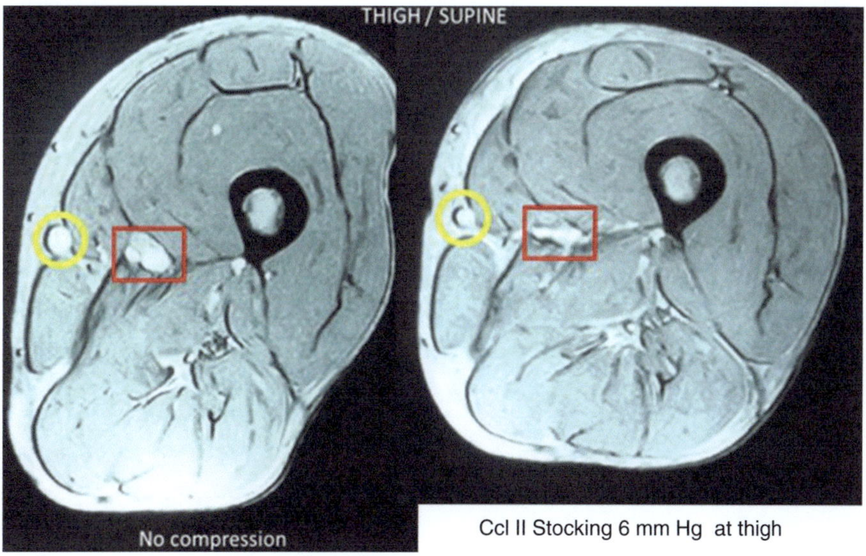

Fig. 2.8 MRI-cross section of a thigh without (left) compression and under a TPS stocking exerting 6 mmHg over this thigh segment (right) [46]

(e.g. stroke) more harm than positive effects have been observed, especially due to not ideally fitting stockings [47]. Nowadays thrombosis prevention is dominated by anticoagulation. However, there is still a good indication for TPS, especially in cases with increased risk of DVT in whom anticoagulants are contraindicated [48].

2.4.2 Compression After Ablation of Varicose Veins

Compression regimes after treatments for varicose veins vary significantly [49].

Adequate compression reduces pain and hematoma formation after surgical removal of varicose veins and after sclerotherapy and all kinds of catheter ablation. Especially eccentric compression using pads for the first postoperative week to increase the local pressure of a treated vein is very effective concerning subjective feelings of the patients [50, 51]. No effects concerning the objective outcome of varicose vein treatment has been observed [52].

2.4.3 Leg-Ulcers, Lipodermatosclerosis

Compression therapy is still the most important form of managing severe stages of chronic venous insufficiency and leg ulcers [53] (see Fig. 2.9).

The main effects of compression are the reduction of venous hypertension using adequate pressure and the anti-inflammatory action.

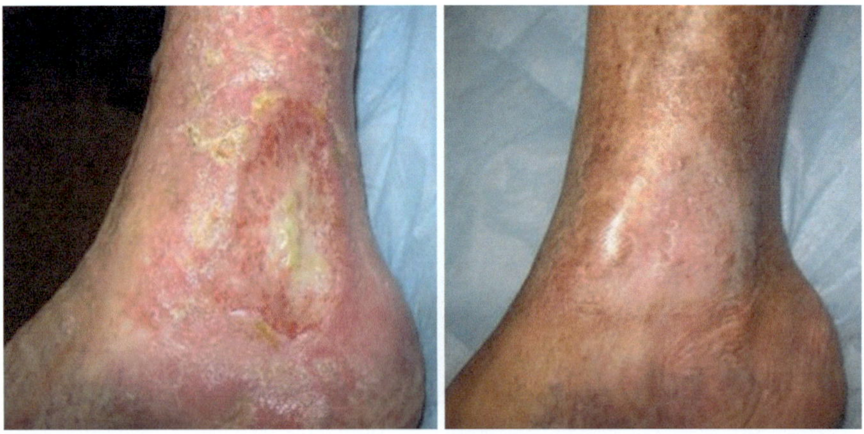

Fig. 2.9 Venous leg ulcer before and after 10 weeks inelastic compression bandages with additional application of rubber foam pads over the ulcer area to increase local pressure following the law of Laplace

2.4.3.1 Reduction of Venous Hypertension

Several clinical studies have shown that compression therapy is able to improve the pumping function of the calf and to reduce ambulatory venous hypertension, provided the compression pressure is high enough to narrow incompetent leg veins in the upright position. As explained above, this is only the case if inelastic material is used exerting a pressure in standing of more than 60–70 mmHg. In this case the peak pressures during walking will block the venous reflux during muscle systole which will decrease the intravenous systolic pressure peaks, even in patients with a complete absence of valves [24]. Measuring the ejection fraction of the calf pump by plethysmography it could be shown that inelastic bandages applied with high pressures were significantly more effective compared to compression stockings [53].

2.4.3.2 Anti-Inflammatory Action

Elevated levels of D-dimer, interleukin-6 (IL-6), and -8 (IL-8), and C- reactive protein (CRP) levels were shown in varicose vein blood taken from foot veins in the standing position in patients with venous insufficiency, compared with upper extremity blood samples [54].

Increased venous pressure leads to increased leucocyte infiltration and abnormal fibroblast function. The extravasation of proteins and iron triggers the inflammatory response, leading to edema, hyperpigmentation, lipodermatosclerosis, and venous ulceration.

Compression improves these mechanisms by an increase of the flow velocity in the microcirculation leading to endothelial neutrophil detachment and reduces elevated levels of the inflammatory cytokines, vascular endothelial growth factor and tumor necrosis factor-in patients with venous ulcers [55, 56].

Lipodermatosclerosis (CEAP C4) or leg ulcers (including those who are not associated with venous incompetence) are good indications for compression therapy, which is also quite effective to reduce pain and swelling in acute superficial and deep vein thrombosis, especially when strongly applied inelastic material is used. The anti-inflammatory action will also have an influence on remodeling of the vein wall, which is one mechanism of action to reduce PTS- in addition to reopening of occluded venous segments. Well-designed clinical studies starting in the acute phase of DVT using strong compression will be necessary to clarify the present debated level of evidence concerning a reduction of PTS by compression [57, 58].

Compression is also very effective in cases with purpura and vasculitis. Erysipelas (cellulitis) is still considered to be a contraindication for compression in several guidelines. As a matter of fact, starting inelastic compression with reduced pressure (“modified compression”) will lead to a fast reduction of edema and pain so that patients are able to get mobile much faster as soon as the fever has subsided in response to antibiotic therapy [59].

2.4.4 Occupational Edema, Dependency Syndrome

Compression is not just a symptomatic form of treatment, since ongoing edema predisposes to inflammation and infection, leads to difficulties in the fitting of clothing and footwear, alters activities of daily life, reduces self-esteem and adversely impacts quality of life. Compression is very effective in preventing and reducing edema. This has been shown in various publications dealing with occupational edema [60] or with leg swelling after long flights, which may occur in otherwise healthy persons. Also, subjective symptoms like tiredness or feeling of heaviness may be reduced. It could be shown that even very light compression pressure of less than 10 mmHg ("placebo stockings") is able to reduce occupational edema [60].

Prolonged sitting in immobile patients, e.g. in those spending their daily life in wheelchairs is one of the most common causes for "chronic edema".

2.4.5 Chronic Edema Due to Systemic Disorders

Chronic edema, which has been defined by leg swelling present for more than 6 weeks, is a very frequent clinical problem, which is often overlooked, or disregarded. Due to the newly discovered fact that the fluid filtrate in the tissue is not reabsorbed by venules as this was taught previously but needs to be transported by the lymphatics [61] every chronic edema may be categorized as lymphedema. The underlying causes are covering a wide range of pathologies which need to be differentiated and treated. Cases in whom excessive production of tissue fluid needs to be overcome by initially still functioning lymphatic drainage which later decompensates must be differentiated from forms with underlying lymphatic damage.

Systemic edema due to incapability of absorbing and transporting excess tissue fluid which is being produced.

Examples for systemic causes which will lead to bilateral swelling, are listed below:

- heart failure
- kidney disease
- hypoproteinemia
- pulmonary hypertension
- hypothyroidism (myxedema)
- Lipedema
- Drug induced
- Dependency syndrome
- Hormonal "cyclic" edema, Morbid obesity

Compression is an important basic treatment modality in all these entities. However, some cases of chronic edema may be cured by removing the underlying cause (e.g. gastric bypass in obese patients, reopening of iliac vein occlusions by a STENT).

2.4.5.1 Is Compression Indicated in Cardiac Insufficiency?

Strong compression of both legs may lead to a shift of blood volume towards the central body regions and may increase the cardiac preload. This is the reason why cardiac insufficiency is clinically considered a contraindication for compression in severe heart failure (NYHA III_IV). Experiments show that compression stockings may further increase the increased values of human natriuretic peptides in patients with heart failure (NYHA II), but only for a short period of time [62].

Strong or high grade compression of both legs should be avoided until the patient's hemodynamic status is stable. It is advisable to start compression with initially low pressures when the patient can get out of bed.

2.4.6 Chronic Venous Insufficiency, Postthrombotic Syndrome (Venous Edema)

Edema due to venous insufficiency is the most frequent indication for compression therapy. For the acute stage of DVT or SVT we start with high pressure bandages and switch to compression stockings to maintain edema reduction that has been achieved in the initial treatment phase. Due to the instant improvement of pain patients can walk better [58]. The combination of high pressure peaks during walking, creating a massage effect seems to be responsible for a faster reopening of the occluded veins in addition to the anti-inflammatory effects on the vein wall, thereby reducing the development severe stages of a PTS.

Venous leg ulcers are the most severe form of chronic venous insufficiency, leading to venous hypertension, caused by persisting vein obstructions and/or by insufficiency of vein valves. In addition to the anti- edematous effect, adequate compression exerts hemodynamic effects reducing ambulatory venous hypertension and is therefore the first method of choice to treat venous leg ulcers [63]. During the last years it could be demonstrated that additional correction of the underlying pathology by reopening of impaired venous outflow in the pelvis and/or abolition of venous reflux may have additional benefits [63]. However, when the ulcer is healed most patients will need continuation of compression, mostly by compression stockings.

2.4.7 Lymphoedema (Failure of Lymphatics)

Lymphedema may be caused by genetic defects of the lymphatic system or by obstruction of the main lymphatics following bacterial inflammation, mechanical trauma, excision of lymph nodes with afferent lymphatics and local irradiation in cancer therapy [64]. Life-long compression therapy is the basis of therapy. Chronic edema and lymphoedema need continuous compression. When compression is discontinued, edema will recur. This is also true after liposuction and other surgical procedures.

Conservative treatment of lymphedema is usually based on "complex decongestion therapy" (CDT) consisting of compression, manual lymph drainage, exercises and skin-care. Compression is the most important component which cannot be replaced by any other method.

We differentiate between a so-called therapy phase and a maintenance phase. The initial therapy phase should start by using compression bandages adjusted to the underlying pathology and limb size [65, 66].

2.4.7.1 Therapy Phase

Inelastic bandages applied by trained personnel staying day and night or Velcro devices should not impede joint movement and avoid slipping. Renewal time needs to be adjusted to the amount of edema reduction (pressure fall) and local facilities. The application of bandages need considerable skill of the bandager. In deformed extremities it resembles the work of a sculptor especially in severe cases. Toes and fingers also need compression to prevent fluid accumulation and papillomatosis.

Short stretch, material will create a massaging effect during exercise which should be encouraged.

Figure 2.10 shows an example in which compression could not only reduce leg circumference but also papillomas.

We recommend an initial resting pressure of the inelastic compression material of around 30 mmHg on the upper and 60 mmHg on the lower extremity [67].

2.4.7.2 Maintaining Limb Volume

When no more volume reduction can be achieved the decongested state should be maintained by further compression which can be performed by the patients themselves, either by made to measure compression stockings (sleeves) or by Velcro devices.

Especially for am lymphedema some experts recommend wearing a sleeve during the day and a compression bandage or a Velcro-device at night during the maintenance phase.

The objective of bandaging can also be to help maintain limb volume reduction or prevent swelling worsening. Flat knit material is preferred because of its higher stiffness (stronger massaging effect) [65]. Stockings usually need to be renewed at least twice a year. New models of Velcro- devices (e.g. Juxta cure©) can be tailored to the individual leg circumferences and used after considerable volume reduction has been achieved [20]. Pressure pumps (Intermittent pneumatic pressure, IPC) are a useful adjunct in both treatment phases which can be helpful especially in patients with restricted mobility, it is discussed in detail in Chap. 11 in this book.

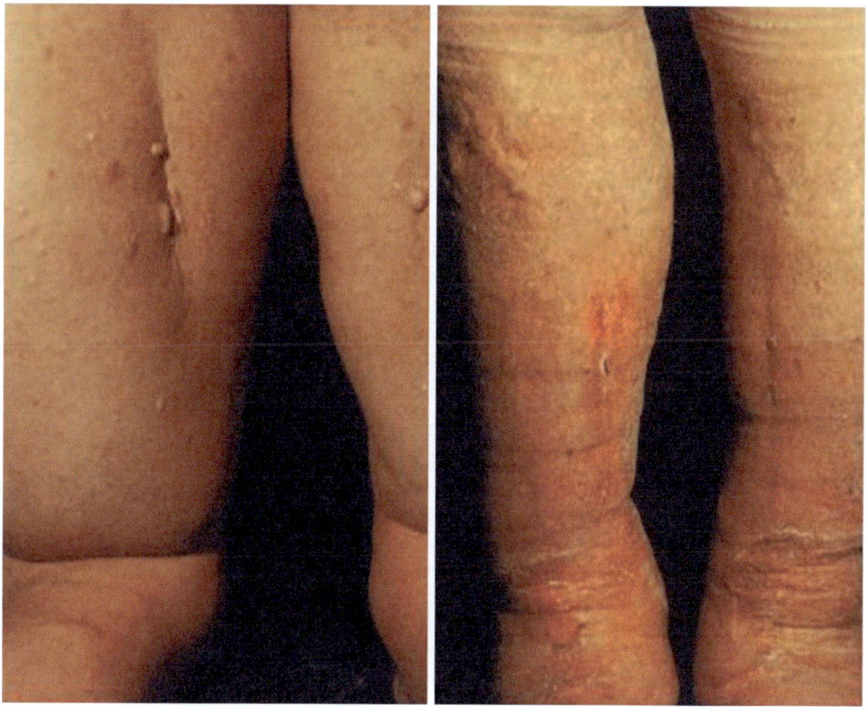

Fig. 2.10 4 weeks of inelastic bandages led to a reduction of swelling and of lymph papillomas in a case of bilateral congenital lymphedema

Additional manual lymph-drainage is helpful especially in the therapy phase but should always be accompanied by acute compression.

The main aims of compression therapy can be summarized as follows [68]:

1. Decrease swelling
2. Increase lymph drainage from the congested areas
3. Reduce skin fibrosis and improve the skin condition
4. Enhance patient's functional status
5. Relieve discomfort and improve quality of life
6. Reduce the risk of cellulitis and malignant transformation.

2.4.8 *Compression in Non-vascular Indications*

Compression therapy has been used traditionally also for several other indications, especially after different kinds of trauma, including bone fractures, to reduce pain and hematoma formation, to stabilize joints or reduce scar formation (keloids) and to manage swelling in cases of Klippel Trenaunay Syndrome [59].

References

1. Thomas S. The production and measurement of sub-bandage pressure: Laplace's Law revisited. J Wound Care. 2014;23(5):234–6, 38–41.
2. Partsch H, Mosti G, Schuren J, Benigni JP. The static stiffness index: an important parameter to characterise compression therapy in vivo. J Wound Care. 2016;25(Suppl 9):S4–S10.
3. Partsch H. Compression for the management of venous leg ulcers: which material do we have? Phlebology. 2014;29(1 suppl):140–5.
4. Neumann HA, Partsch H, Mosti G, Flour M. Classification of compression stockings: report of the meeting of the International Compression Club,Copenhagen. Int Angiol. 2016;35(2):122–8.
5. Partsch H, Clark M, Bassez S, Benigni JP, Becker F, et al. Measurement of lower leg compression in vivo: recommendations for the performance of measurements of interface pressure and stiffness: consensus statement. Dermatol Surg. 2006;32(2):224–32.
6. Partsch H, Mosti G. Comparison of three portable instruments to measure compression pressure. Int Angiol. 2010;29(5):426–30.
7. Partsch H, Clark M, Mosti G, Steinlechner E, Schuren J, et al. Classification of compression bandages: practical aspects. Dermatol Surg. 2008;34(5):600–9.
8. Stolk R, Wegen van der-Franken CP, Neumann HA. A method for measuring the dynamic behavior of medical compression hosiery during walking. Dermatol Surg. 2004;30(5):729–36.
9. CEN. Comité Européen de Normalisation. 2001:1–40. Located at: European Prestandard. Medical compression hosiery. European Committee for Standardization, Brussels.
10. Partsch H. The use of pressure change on standing as a surrogate measure of the stiffness of a compression bandage. Eur J Vasc Endovasc Surg. 2005;30(4):415–21.
11. Sigel B, Edelstein AL, Savitch L, et al. Type of compression for reducing venous stasis. A study of lower extremities during inactive recumbency. Arch Surg. 1975;110:171–5.
12. Murthy G, Ballard RE, Breit GA, Watenpaugh DE, Hargens AR. Intramuscular pressures beneath elastic and inelastic leggings. Ann Vasc Surg. 1994;8(6):543–8.
13. Flour M, Clark M, Partsch H, Mosti G, Uhl JF, et al. Dogmas and controversies in compression therapy: report of an International Compression Club (ICC) meeting, Brussels, May 2011. Int Wound J. 2013;10(5):516–26.
14. Mosti G, Partsch H. Compression stockings with a negative pressure gradient have a more pronounced effect on venous pumping function than graduated elastic compression stockings. Eur J Vasc Endovasc Surg. 2011;42(2):261–6.
15. Mosti G, Partsch H. Improvement of venous pumping function by double progressive compression stockings: higher pressure over the calf is more important than a graduated pressure profile. Eur J Vasc Endovasc Surg. 2014;47(5):545–9.
16. Sippel K, Seifert B, Hafner J. Donning devices (foot slips and frames) enable elderly people with severe chronic venous insufficiency to put on compressionstockings. Eur J Vasc Endovasc Surg. 2015;49(2):221–9.
17. Luder C, Dziunycz P, Omid N, Radetzki AL, Lang C, Hübner M, Hafner J. A Compression Kit of a Stocking and Three Superimposed Leggings Is Easy to Don and Dose Adjustable. Eur J Vasc Endovasc Surg. 2016;51(3):434–40.
18. Heyer K, Protz K, Augustin M. Compression therapy—cross-sectional observational survey about knowledge and practical treatment of specialised and non-specialised nurses and therapists. Int Wound J. 2017;14(6):1148–53.
19. Zarchi K, Jemec GB. Delivery of compression therapy for venous leg ulcers. JAMA Dermatol. 2014;150(7):730–6.
20. Damstra RJ, Partsch H. Prospective, randomized, controlled trial comparing the effectiveness of adjustable compression Velcro wraps versus inelastic multicomponent compression bandages in the initial treatment of leg lymphedema. J Vasc Surg Venous Lymphat Disord. 2013;1(1):13–9.
21. Ludbrook J. Aspects of venous function in the lower limbs. Springfield, IL: Charles C. Thomas; 1968.

22. Partsch B, Partsch H. Calf compression pressure required to achieve venous closure from supine to standing positions. J Vasc Surg. 2005;42(4):734–8.
23. Partsch H. Improving the venous pumping function in chronic venous insufficiency by compression as dependent on pressure and material. Vasa. 1984;13(1):58–64.
24. Partsch B, Mayer W, Partsch H. Improvement of ambulatory venous hypertension by Narrowing of the Femoral Vein in Congenital Absence of Venous Valves. Phlebology. 1992;7: 101–4.
25. Mayrovitz HN, Larsen PB. Effects of compression bandaging on leg pulsatile blood flow. Clin Physiol. 1997;17(1):105–17.
26. Jünger M, Haase H, Schwenke L, Bichel J, Schuren J, Ladwig A. Macro- and microperfusion during application of a new compression system, designed for patients with leg ulcer and concomitant peripheral arterial occlusive disease. Clin Hemorheol Microcirc. 2013;53(3): 281–93.
27. Mosti G, Iabichella ML, Partsch H. Compression therapy in mixed ulcers increases venous output and arterial perfusion. J Vasc Surg. 2012;55(1):122–8.
28. Zaki M, Elsherif M, Tawfick W, El Sharkawy M, Hynes N, Sultan S. The role of sequential pneumatic compression in limb salvage in non- reconstructable critical limb ischemia. Eur J Vasc Endovasc Surg. 2016;51(4):565–71.
29. Buschmann EE, Brix M, Li L, Doreen J, Zietzer A, Li M, Buschmann I, Hillmeister P. Adaptation of external counterpulsation based on individual shear rate therapy improves endothelial function and claudication distance in peripheral artery disease. Vasa. 2016;45(4):317–24.
30. Chen AH, Frangos SG, Kilaru S, Sumpio BE. Intermittent pneumatic compression devices – physiological mechanisms of action. Eur J Vasc Endovasc Surg. 2001 May;21(5):383–92.
31. Mani R. Transcutaneous measurements of oxygen tension in venous ulcer disease. Vasc Med Rev. 1995;6:121–31.
32. Bollinger A, Fagrell B. Clinical capillaroscopy. Toronto: Hofgreve & Huber Publishers; 1990.
33. Abu-Own A, Cheatle T, Scurr JH, Coleridge Smith PD. Effects of intermittent pneumatic compression of the foot on the microcirculatory function in arterial disease. Eur J Vasc Surg. 1993;7(5):488–92.
34. Barnes M, Mani R, Barrett DF, White JE. Changes in skin microcirculation at periulcerous sites in patients with chronic venous ulcers during leg elevation. Phlebology. 1992;7:36–9.
35. Bakker K, Apelqvist JAP, Schaper NC. Practical guidelines on the management and prevention of the diabetic foot. Diabetes Metab Res Rev. 2012;28(S1):30–5.
36. Mathieu D. Mani R. A review of the clinical significance of tissue hypoxia measurements in lower extremity wound management. Int J Low Extremity. Wounds. 2007;6(4):273–83.
37. Olszewski WL, Engeset A. Intrinsic contractility of prenodal lymph vessels and lymph flow in human leg. Am J Phys. 1980;239(6):H775–83.
38. Olszewski WL. Contractility patterns of normal and pathologically changed human lymphatics. Ann N Y Acad Sci. 2002;979:52–63.
39. Breslin JW. Mechanical forces and lymphatic transport. Microvasc Res. 2014;96:46–54.
40. Lahtinen T, Seppälä J, Viren T, Johansson K. Experimental and analytical comparisons of tissue dielectric constant (TDC) and bioimpedance spectroscopy (BIS) in assessment of early arm lymphedema in breast cancer patients after axillary surgery and radiotherapy. Lymphat Res Biol. 2015;13(3):176–85.
41. Zaleska M, Olszewski WL, Cakala M, Cwikla J, Budlewski T. Intermittent pneumatic compression enhances formation of edema tissue fluid channels in lymphedema of lower limbs. Lymphat Res Biol. 2015;13(2):146–53.
42. Zaleska M, Olszewski WL, Durlik M, Kaczmarek M. A novel clinical test for setting intermittent pneumatic compression parameters based on edema fluid hydromechanics in the lymphedematous Calf. Lymphat Res Biol. 2015;13(3):208–14.
43. Kakkar VV. A physiological study of elastic compression stockings in venous disorders of the leg. Phlebologie. 1982;35(1):101–6.
44. Partsch H. Compression therapy: clinical and experimental evidence. Ann Vasc Dis. 2012;5(4):416–22.

45. Downie SP, Raynor SM, Firmin DN, Wood NB, Thom SA, et al. Effects of elastic compression stockings on wall shear stress in deep and superficial veins of the calf. Am J Physiol Heart Circ Physiol. 2008;294(5):H2112–20.
46. Partsch H, Mosti G, Mosti F. Narrowing of leg veins under compression demonstrated by magnetic resonance imaging (MRI). Int Angiol. 2010;29(5):408–10.
47. Dennis M, Sandercot PA, Reid J, et al. The CLOTS Trials Collaboration. Effectiveness of thigh-length graduated compression stockings to reduce the risk of deep vein thrombosis after stroke (CLOTS trial 1): a multicentre, randomised controlled trial. Lancet. 2009;373:1958–65.
48. Nicolaides AN, Breddin HK, Carpenter P, Coccheri S, Conard J, et al. Thrombophilia and venous thromboembolism. International consensus statement. Guidelines according to scientific evidence. Int Angiol. 2005;24(1):1–26.
49. El-Sheikha J, Nandhra S, Carradice D, Acey C, Smith GE, et al. Compression regimes after endovenous ablation for superficial venous insufficiency – a survey of members of the Vascular Society of Great Britain and Ireland. Phlebology. 2016;31(1):16–22.
50. Lugli M, Cogo A, Guerzoni S, Petti A, Maleti O. Effects of eccentric compression by a crossed-tape technique after endovenous laser ablation of thegreat saphenous vein: a randomized study. Phlebology. 2009;24(4):151–6.
51. Mosti G, Mattaliano V, Arleo S, Partsch H. Thigh compression after great saphenous surgery is more effective with high pressure. Int Angiol. 2009;28(4):274–80.
52. Rabe E, Partsch H, Hafner J, Lattimer C, Mosti G, et al. Indications for medical compression stockings in venous and lymphatic disorders: An evidence-based consensus statement. Phlebology. 2018;33(3):163–84.
53. Mosti G, Mattaliano V, Partsch H. Inelastic compression increases venous ejection fraction more than elastic bandages in patients with superficial venous reflux. Phlebology. 2008;23(6):287–94.
54. Lattimer CR, Ligi D, Mannello F, Kalodiki E. Effect of compression and lying down on local MMPs from the dependent leg in healthy subjects & varicose vein patients. Presentation at the 30thAnnual Meeting of the AVF, Tucson AZ Feb 20–23. J Vasc Surg. In press.
55. Murphy MA, Joyce WP, Condron C, Bouchier-Hayes D. A reduction in serum cytokine levels parallels healing of venous ulcers in patients undergoing compression therapy. Eur J Endovasc Surg. 2002;23:349–52.
56. Beidler SK, Douillet CD, Berndt DF, Keagy BA, Rich PB, Marston WA. Inflammatory cytokine levels in chronic venous insufficiency ulcer tissue before and after compression therapy. J Vasc Surg. 2009;49(4):1013–20.
57. Ten Cate-Hoek AJ, Amin EE, Bouman AC, Meijer K, Tick LW, et al. IDEAL DVT investigators. Individualised versus standard duration of elastic compression therapy for prevention of post-thrombotic syndrome (IDEAL DVT): a multicentre, randomised, single-blind, allocation-concealed, non-inferiority trial. Lancet Haematol 2018;5(1):e25–33.
58. Partsch H. The role of leg compression in the treatment of deep vein thrombosis. Phlebology. 2014;29(1 suppl):66–70. Epub 2014 May 19.
59. Cinderella indications for compression - International Compression Club (ICC) Meeting, 2015. http://www.pagepressjournals.org/index.php/vl/issue/view/414.
60. Partsch H, Winiger J, Lun B. Compression stockings reduce occupational leg swelling. Dermatol Surg. 2004;30(5):737–43.
61. Levick JR. Revision of the Starling principle: new views of tissue fluid balance. J Physiol. 2004;557(Pt 3):704.
62. Galm O, Jansen-Genzel W, von Helden J, Wienert V. Plasma human atrial natriuretic peptide under compression therapy in patients with chronic venous insufficiency with or without cardiac insufficiency. Vasa. 1996;25(1):48–53.
63. O'Donnell TF Jr, Passman MA, Marston WA, Ennis WJ, Dalsing M, et al. Society for Vascular Surgery; AmericanVenous Forum. Management of venous leg ulcers: clinical practice guidelines of the Society for Vascular Surgery ® and the American Venous Forum. J Vasc Surg. 2014;60(2 Suppl):3S–59S.

64. Földi M, Földi E, Kubik S. Textbook of lymphology. München: Urban & Fischer; 2003.
65. International Lymph network position Document: best practice for the management of lymphoedema, 2nd ed. https://www.lympho.org/wp-content/uploads/2016/03/Compression-bandaging-final.pdf.
66. Lee BB, Rockson SG, Bergan J, editors. Lymphedema A concise compendium of theory and practice. New York: Springer; 2018.
67. Partsch H, Damstra RJ, Mosti G. Dose finding for an optimal compression pressure to reduce chronic edema of the extremities. Int Angiol. 2011;30(6):527–33.
68. Position Statement of the National Lymphedema Network. http://www.strengthandcourage.net/pdfs/Lymphedema%20and%20Exercise.pdf.

Chapter 3
Delivering Compression to Treat Chronic Wounds in the UK & Ireland

Georgina Gethin and Andrew Ross Cameron

Abstract Consensus opinion and systematic reviews supports the use of compression therapy as the 'gold standard' for the management of venous leg ulceration (VLU). However, although widely used, significant limitations to this treatment modality persist including; poor compliance, negative impact on quality of life, bandage bulk limiting footwear choices, high visibility to others, cost and the requirement in most cases for application by health care professionals. Additionally, based on results of over 48 RCTs healing outcomes are improved with compression, yet, overall healing rates leave significant scope for improvement. This chapter describes the various systems available in the United Kingdom and Ireland together with the indications and limitations for use.

Keywords Compression · Venous ulceration · Contraindications · ABPI · Compliance · Healing

3.1 The Benefits of Compression Therapy for Treatment of Chronic Wounds

Within the UK and Ireland, compression therapy forms an integral part of the clinical gold standard treatment for chronic wounds stemming from venous or lymphatic insufficiency. In the treatment of venous leg ulcers (VLUs) for example, compression therapy is designed to overcome venous insufficiency by providing an external force that works in concert with the body's natural pump functions, such as the contraction and relaxation of the calf muscle, to promote venous return. While there is some debate as to the most effective form of compression therapy [1], there is consensus that compression therapy is better than non-compression [2, 3] and

G. Gethin (✉)
National University of Ireland Galway, Galway, Ireland
e-mail: georgina.gethin@nuigalway.ie

A. R. Cameron
The University of Queensland, St Lucia, QLD, Australia

R. Mani et al. (eds.), *Compression and Chronic Wound Management*,
https://doi.org/10.1007/978-3-030-01195-6_3

different forms of compression can have similarly high rates of successful treatment when used correctly in experienced hands.

3.2 Prevalence of Wounds and Conditions Requiring Compression Therapy

It is estimated the lifetime prevalence of VLUs in the total Western population is 1%, with people aged 65 years and older having a prevalence of 3–4% [2, 3]. Within the United Kingdom (UK), the annual incidence of VLUs in the adult population is 0.59% or approximately 278,000 patients per year [4]. Of those patients with VLUs (which make up 70–90% of all leg ulcer patients [2, 5]), approximately 10% of patients will not benefit from compression therapy as it does not address other underlying pathologies including foot pump insufficiency, lipodermatosclerosis, chronic venous compartment syndrome or non-re-canalized thrombosis [6]. Moreover, of the 15–30% of patients with mixed arteriovenous ulcers (i.e. ABPI < 0.85) [7–9], approximately 15% have an ABPI of <0.5, which is clinically contraindicated for compression therapy [10]. Even after excluding these inapplicable or contraindicated patients, there remains approximately 240,000 VLU patients within the UK who can benefit from compression therapy each year.

In addition to VLU treatment, compression therapy is also the gold standard treatment in Ireland and the UK for other indications such as lymphedema and chronic oedema [11]. Lymphedema is a progressive chronic condition that causes tissue swelling due to malformation (primary lymphedema) or damage to the lymphatic drainage system (secondary lymphedema). Like the treatment of VLUs, it is important to apply a designated level of pressure when treating lymphedema with compression, depending on the severity of swelling or the phase of treatment (e.g. intensive versus maintenance) [12]. While UK based studies have shown the incidence of primary lymphedema is low at approximately 1:2763 to 1:5719, the general prevalence of lymphoedema in these regions is much higher at 2.29–3.59 per 1000 population [13]. These rates of prevalence are similar to those of chronic oedema patients in the UK, with one recent study finding the crude prevalence of chronic oedema in Derby City to be 3.93 per 1000 population [14].

The profile of people with VLUs is one of multi-morbidity and living with a chronic, recurrent condition in what has been described as a body that cannot be trusted. The literature suggests that people with a VLU have an average age of 60–69 years with females more frequently affected in a ratio of 2:1. Furthermore, 23–68% have hypertension [15, 16], 16–48.5% have diabetes [15, 16], approximately 33% are obese with a BMI >30 [16, 17], one third have 3+ co-morbidities [16, 17], and 42–66% have problems with mobility [15, 16]. The health related quality of life for those living with a VLU has been well reported with the most frequent issues being pain, fear of recurrence or further injury, isolation and odour [18, 19]. These issues, while improving once an ulcer has healed, often remain long-term, and for some patients, other problems that remain unaddressed include sleep problems (73%), footwear (70%) and coping with the negative effects of compression (71%) [16, 20].

3.3 Burden of Wound Care to Healthcare Systems

The significant rates of chronic wounds within the UK and Ireland provide a substantial burden to the respective health care systems. Studies have shown that in some areas of Ireland, up to 66% of community nurses' time is spent dealing with wound care [21]. Another recent study has shown the cost of treating VLUs in UK is approximately £7600 per ulcer (£2981 per VLU for the 53% of cases that heal within 12 months and £13,455 per VLU for the 47% of cases unhealed within 12 months) [22]. Overall, the average annual cost to the NHS for management of VLUs, after adjustment for comorbidities, is between £596.6 and £921.9 million [4]. While results from some large scale Canadian trials have shown VLU healing rates as high as 93% after 12 months of compression treatment [23], others from the UK have been as low as 55% [24], and it is known that healing rates can be lower in UK community settings compared to those in specialty clinics [25]. Therefore, the correct application of appropriate compression therapy may represent a means of reducing the economic burden of wound care to the healthcare systems in the UK and Ireland.

3.4 Different Forms of Compression

There are a large variety of compression therapy products available within the UK and Irish healthcare systems, which offer different degrees and different forms of compression based on their inherent properties and functionality. Broadly speaking, compression therapy products can be categorised as compression bandages (e.g. single- or multi-layer bandages that are applied to a limb in a spiral fashion), compression hosiery (e.g. elastic stockings or sleeves), or compression devices (e.g. adjustable Velcro wraps (AVWs) or intermittent pneumatic compression devices). While intermittent pneumatic compression is commonly used in the USA for treatment of lymphoedema and symptomatic venous disorders [26], this compression modality is not routinely used in the treatment of chronic wounds in the UK or Ireland and will not be covered in this Chapter. Figure 3.1 outlines examples of the variations in product properties that comprise the different modalities of compression therapy, including properties related to elasticity, pressure applied, layering, actuation, materials, and material architectures.

Table 3.1 lists the different compression therapies that are currently available on formulary for the treatment of wounds within the UK and Irish healthcare systems, including compression bandages, compression hosiery, and compression

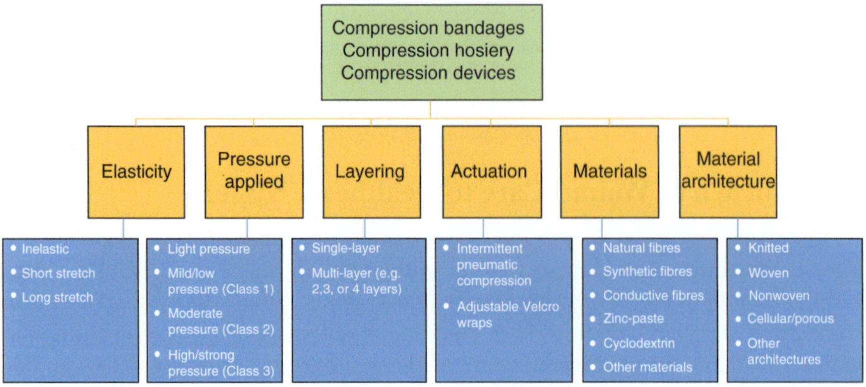

Fig. 3.1 Variations in product properties that comprise the different modalities of compression therapy (adapted from [27])

devices. It should be noted that a substantial number of other compression hosiery products are indicated specifically for lymphoedema, however these have not been listed as lymphoedema specific compression is outside the scope of this Chapter. It should also be noted that specific contraindications for each product are not mentioned in detail, however compression therapies are generally problematic and should be used with a high degree of caution in patients with arterial disease (e.g. peripheral arterial occlusive disease), cardiac disease (e.g. decompensated cardiac insufficiency), severe infection (e.g. septic phlebitis), or large venous blood clots (e.g. phlegmasia coerulea dolens). Some bandages are also not suitable for people with smaller circumference legs (e.g. <18 cm) because of the potential for high pressure application due to high radius of curvature and bony prominences [28]. When indicated by the manufacturer, Table 3.1 lists the ABPI range for a product, but as a general practice, compression therapy is only provided to patients with an ABPI between 0.5 and 0.8 if it is under supervision, and with regular follow-up. While compression therapy has been shown to be beneficial to patients with mixed aetiology ulcers [29–31], it is absolutely contraindicated for patients with an ABPI <0.5.

3.5 Compression Bandages

When determining the most appropriate form of compression therapy to apply to a wound, an internationally recognised standard classification system is used for categorising chronic venous disorders. The CEAP classification system [32, 33] characterises the disease state according to the clinical class (C) based upon objective signs, the aetiology (E), the anatomical (A) distribution of reflux/obstruction in the venous system, and the underlying pathophysiology (P), including whether venous

Table 3.1 Compression bandage, compression hosiery (leg ulceration), and compression device products on the UK and Irish healthcare formulary

Product (Company)	Description	Indications	ABPI range	No. of sizes	Cost range
Compression bandages: Single-layer bandages (SLB)					
Coban Self-Adherent Wrap (3M)	SLB E	• Compression/ support/secure dressings	DNM	1	£2.93
Atico (L&R)	SLB SS	• VLU • Lymphedema • CO	0.8–1.3 (>1.3 requires further investigation)	5	£2.44–4.34
Clinistretch Short (Haddenham Healthcare)	SLB SS	• Varicosis • Chronic venous insufficiency • VLU • Lymphedema (primary and secondary) • Thrombophlebitis • DVT • Post-surgery	DNM	4	£2.65–4.20
Comprilan (BSN medical)	SLB SS	• Varicosis • Chronic venous insufficiency • VLU • Lymphedema (primary and secondary) • Thrombophlebitis • DVT • Post-surgery	DNM	4	£2.72–4.19
K-Plus (Urgo Medical)	SLB E	• VLU (20 mmHg)	≥0.8	2	£2.31–2.67
K-ThreeC (Urgo Medical)	SLB E	• VLU (25–35 mmHg)	≥0.8	1	£2.87
Ko-Flex (Urgo Medical)	SLB E	• VLU (20 mmHg) • Support for limbs after sprains/ strains • Post-surgery rehabilitation	≥0.8	2	£3.07–3.51
Rosidal K (L&R)	SLB SS	• VLU • Lymphoedema	≥0.8	5	£2.67–6.07
Setopress (Molnlycke Health Care)	SLB E	• VLU	DNM	1	£3.58
Tensopress (BSN medical)	SLB E	• VLU	DNM	2	£2.73–3.51

(continued)

Table 3.1 (continued)

Product (Company)	Description	Indications	ABPI range	No. of sizes	Cost range
Compression bandages: Multi-layer bandages (MLB)					
Coban 2 Compression System (3M)	MLB [2]	• VLU • Lymphedema • CO (lower limbs, hips, torso)	≥0.8	Layer 1: 4 Layer 2: 3	Layer 1: £2.86–13.26 Layer 2: £1.43–7.14
Coban 2 Compression System Kit (3M)	MLB [2]	• VLU • Lymphedema • CO	≥0.8	Layer 1: 4 Layer 2: 3	£8.24
Coban 2 Lite Compression System (3M)	MLB [2]	• VLU • Lymphedema • CO (arms, shoulders, fingers, toes)	≥0.8	Layer 1: 3 Layer 2: 4	Layer 1: £4.69–8.77 Layer 2: £2.24–6.22
Coban 2 Lite Compression System Kit (3M)	MLB [2]	• VLU • Lymphedema • CO (arms, shoulders, fingers, toes)	≥0.8	Layer 1: 3 Layer 2: 4	£8.24
Atico 2C (L&R)	MLB [2]	• VLU • CO	0.8–1.3 (unless specialist referral)	2	£8.08–9.10
AndoFlex TLC XL with Malodour Control 2 Layer Kit (Aspen Medical Europe)	MLB [2] Includes cyclodextrin for malodour control	• Malodorous VLU • Misshapen limbs	>0.8	1	£8.45
AndoFlex UBZ 2 Layer Kit With Zinc (Aspen Medical Europe)	MLB [2] Includes zinc for skin irritation	• VLU	>0.8	2	£5.25–6.35
AndoFlex TLC Lite with Malodour Control 10 cm 2 Layer Kit (Aspen Medical Europe)	MLB [2] Includes cyclodextrin for malodour control	• Malodorous VLU	>0.5	1	£7.20

Table 3.1 (continued)

Product (Company)	Description	Indications	ABPI range	No. of sizes	Cost range
AndoFlex TLC with Malodour Control 10 cm 2 Layer Kit (Aspen Medical Europe)	MLB [2] Includes cyclodextrin for malodour control	• Malodorous VLU	>0.8	1	£7.20
Clinistretch (Haddenham Healthcare)	MLB [2]	• VLU • Lymphedema (lower limbs, arms) • CO (lower limbs, arms)	0.8–1.3 (unless specialist referral)	5	£2.42–4.31
Hero H-2 (H&R Healthcare)	MLB [2] Includes cyclodextrin for malodour control Includes aloe for moisture control	• VLU • MAU	DNM	Kit: 3 Layer 1: 2	Kit: £7.04–8.05 Layer 1: £4.23–4.83
Jobst Compri2 (BSN medical)	MLB [2]	• VLU + oedema • Lymphatic oedema		2	£6.71–7.67
Jobst Compri2 Lite (BSN medical)	MLB [2]	• MAU	0.5–0.8	2	£6.71–8.45
Jobst Comprifore (BSN medical)	MLB [4]	• VLU	≥0.8	1	£6.87
Jobst Comprifore Latex-free (BSN medical)	MLB [4]	• VLU	≥0.8	1	£7.23
Jobst Comprifore Lite (BSN medical)	MLB [3]	• VLU	0.6–0.8	1	£4.49
Jobst Comprifore Lite Latex-free (BSN medical)	MLB [3]	• VLU	0.6–0.8	1	£4.84

(continued)

Table 3.1 (continued)

Product (Company)	Description	Indications	ABPI range	No. of sizes	Cost range
K-Four (Urgo Medical)	MLB [4]	• VLU	≥0.8	4	Kits: £4.55–9.58 Individual layers: £0.46–3.07
Profore (Smith & Nephew)	MLB [4]	• VLU	≥0.8	4	Kits: £8.00–11.99 Individual layers: £0.32–4.00
Profore Lite (Smith & Nephew)	MLB [3]	• VLU	≥0.6	1	Kit: £5.57
Profore Latex Free (Smith & Nephew)	MLB [4]	• VLU	≥0.8	1	Kit: £10.30 Individual layers: £0.77–4.34
Profore Latex Free Lite (Smith & Nephew)	MLB [3]	• VLU	≥0.6	1	Kit: £6.05
Ultra Four (Robinson Healthcare)	MLB [4]	• VLU	DNM	3	Kits: £4.14–6.41 Individual layers: £0.39–2.59
UrgoKTwo (Urgo Medical)	MLB [2]	• VLU • Oedema • Lymphoedema	≥0.8	10	£6.95–11.35
UrgoKTwo Reduced (Urgo Medical)	MLB [2]	• MAU • Oedema • Lymphoedema	≥0.6	4	£8.24–9.56
UrgoKTwo with UrgoStart (Urgo Medical)	MLB [2] Includes polyester contact mesh impregnated with hydrocolloid, petroleum jelly and oligosaccharide.	• Non-infected VLU	≥0.8	2	£10.27–10.95

Table 3.1 (continued)

Product (Company)	Description	Indications	ABPI range	No. of sizes	Cost range
Compression bandages: Padding					
Cellona Undercast Padding (L&R)	Synthetic padding	• For use under SLB	DNM	4	£0.31–0.6
Clinistretch Soft (Haddenham Healthcare)	Wadding bandage	• For use under SLB and casts	DNM	1	£0.47
FlexiBan (L&R)	Bandage padding	• For use under SLB	DNM	1	£0.50
K-Soft (Urgo Medical)	Sub-bandage wadding	• Reducing the effect of compression, reshaping legs/ ankles, protect bony prominences	DNM	2	£0.46–0.58
Rosidal Soft (L&R)	Padding material	• For use under compression bandages	DNM	3	£5.23–8.08
Compression hosiery (leg ulceration): Single layer					
ActiLymph Hosiery Kit (L&R)	Class 2 With liner	• Venous disorders • Oedema • Lymphoedema • VLU • VLU recurrence prevention • Severe varicose veins	0.8–1.3 (unless specialist referral)	5	£30.44
Activa British Standard Compression Hosiery (L&R)	Class 1–3	• Class 1: Early varices, DVT prevention when travelling • Class 2: Medium varices, prevention of VLU • Class 3: Gross varices, treatment and prevention of VLU, post-thrombotic venous insufficiency	0.8–1.3 (unless specialist referral)	Class 1: 4 Class 2: 5 Class 3: 5	£7.58–14.61

(continued)

Table 3.1 (continued)

Product (Company)	Description	Indications	ABPI range	No. of sizes	Cost range
Activa Class 1 Unisex Sock (L&R)	Class 1	• Mild venous disorders • DVT prevention when travelling	0.8–1.3 (unless specialist referral)	4	£7.58
Activa Class 2 Unisex Sock (L&R)	Class 2	• Medium severity venous disorders • Prevention of VLU • DVT prevention when travelling	0.8–1.3 (unless specialist referral)	4	£11.08
Altiform British Standard Compression Hosiery (Urgo Medical)	Class 1–3	• Class 1: Early varices, varicosis during pregnancy • Class 2: Medium varices, treatment and prevention of VLU • Class 3: Gross varices, treatment and prevention of VLU, post-thrombotic venous insufficiency, gross oedema, treatment and prevention of VLU	DNM	Class 1: 4 Class 2: 4 Class 3: 4	£7.89–13.90
Altiform British Standard Made to Measure Compression Hosiery (Urgo Medical)	Class 1–3	• Class 1: Early varices, varicosis during pregnancy • Class 2: Medium varices, treatment and prevention of VLU • Class 3: Gross varices, treatment and prevention of VLU, post-thrombotic venous insufficiency, gross oedema, treatment and prevention of VLU	DNM	Class 1: 1 Class 2: 1 Class 3: 1	£26.46–42.30

Table 3.1 (continued)

Product (Company)	Description	Indications	ABPI range	No. of sizes	Cost range
Carolon Multi-layer Compression System Understocking Pack (H&R Healthcare)	Class I Copper yarn for malodour	• VLU	DNM	7	£22.00
Credalast (Credenhill)	Class 1–3	• Class 1: Early varices, varicosis during pregnancy • Class 2: Medium varices, treatment and prevention of VLU, mild oedema and varicosis during pregnancy • Class 3: Gross varices, treatment and prevention of VLU, post-thrombotic venous insufficiency, gross oedema, treatment and prevention of VLU	DNM	Class 1: 4 Class 2: 4 Class 3: 4	Standard: £7.58–14.61 Made to measure: £27.47–43.91
Duomed Soft – BS Hosiery (medi UK)	Class 1–3	• Class 1: Early varices • Class 2: Medium varices, treatment and prevention of VLU, mild oedema • Class 3: Gross varices, treatment and prevention of VLU, post-thrombotic venous insufficiency, gross oedema, treatment and prevention of VLU	DNM	Class 1: 5 Class 2: 5 Class 3: 5	£7.58–14.61

(continued)

Table 3.1 (continued)

Product (Company)	Description	Indications	ABPI range	No. of sizes	Cost range
Eesilite (Sallis)	Class 1–3	• Class 1: Early varices • Class 2: Medium varices, treatment and prevention of VLU, mild oedema • Class 3: Gross varices, treatment and prevention of VLU, post-thrombotic venous insufficiency, gross oedema, treatment and prevention of VLU	DNM	Class 1: 4 Class 2: 4 Class 3: 4	£7.30–14.08
Premier MTM Ulcer Care Sock (Jobskin)	Class 3 Includes zipper	• VLU	DNM	Custom	Not listed
Venosan 2000 (Credenhill)	Class 2–3	• Chronic venous insufficiency	DNM	Class 2: 4 Class 3: 4	Not listed
Venosan Legline (Credenhill)	Class 1	• Varicosis during pregnancy, support after sclerotherapy	DNM	5	Not listed
Tubular Support Bandages 4214 (Bastos Viegas S.A.)	Tubular support bandages	• Rehabilitation • Support for sprains/strains • Oedema • Joint effusions	DNM	11	£2.93–110.81
Compression hosiery (leg ulceration): Multi-layer hosiery					
Activa Leg Ulcer Hosiery Kits (L&R)	MLH [2]	• Venous disorders • Prevention and management of VLU	0.8–1.3 (unless specialist referral)	5	Kit: £23.09 Liners: £16.97–17.31
Alleviant Ulcer Care Kit (Jobskin)	MLH [2] Silver thread for antimicrobial properties	• Prevention and management of VLU	DNM	7	£30
Altipress 40 Leg Ulcer Kit (AltiMed)	MLH [2]	• VLU	DNM	5	Kit: £14.61 Liners: £11.56

Table 3.1 (continued)

Product (Company)	Description	Indications	ABPI range	No. of sizes	Cost range
Altipress 40 Made to Measure Ulcer Kit (AltiMed)	MLH [2]	• VLU	DNM	Made to order	Kit: £42.39 Liners: £24.01
Carolon Multi-layer Compression System (H&R Healthcare)	MLH [2] Copper yarn for malodour	• VLU (after oedema controlled)	DNM	Black: 5 Beige: 7	£26.50
Clini Duo40 (CliniSupplies)	MLH [2]	• VLU	0.8–1.2	5	Kit: £13.07 Liners: £10.34
Compression Leg Ulcer Kit (Synergy Health)	MLH [2]	• VLU	DNM	5	Kit: £12.45 Liners: £9.85
Jobst UlcerCare (BSN medical)	MLH [2] Includes zipper	• Following oedema reduction by SS bandage	DNM	7	Kit: £31.81 Liner pack: £19.21
Jobst UlcerCare Custom Fit (BSN medical)	MLH [2] Includes zipper	• Following oedema reduction by SS bandage	DNM	Custom	Kit: £64.46 Liner pack: £32.23
medivan ulcer kit (medi UK)	MLH [2]	• VLU	DNM	7	Kit: £32.48 Liner pack: £17.41
Ulcer X Kit and Ulcer X Liners (Sigvaris)	MLH [2]	• VLU	DNM	4	Kit: £24.54 Liner pack: £20.89
Ulcertec (Bauerfeind)	MLH [2]	• VLU	DNM	5	£27.10
Venosan 8000 Ulcerfit (Credenhill)	MLH [2]	• VLU	DNM	Class 2: 4 Class 4: 4	Kit: £21.85 Liner pack: £13.01
Compression devices: Adjustable Velcro wraps (AVWs)					
Haddenham Easywrap (Haddenham Healthcare)	AVW	• Light (20–30 mmHg): Mild-moderate lymphedema and • CO • Strong (30–40 mmHg): Moderate-severe lymphedema and • CO	DNM	Arm: 24 Foot: 10 Leg: 10 Thigh: 10	Arm: £135.46 Hand: £28.09 Foot: £36.12 Leg: £128.93 Thigh: £128.93

(continued)

Table 3.1 (continued)

Product (Company)	Description	Indications	ABPI range	No. of sizes	Cost range
Juxtacures (medi UK)	AVW Built in pressure system guide Designed for 6 months daily use	• VLU	DNM	3	Pack (Juxtacures, 2 anklets, 2 liners): £155.01 Liners: £13.49 Anklets: £11.42
Juxtalite (medi UK)	AVW Built in pressure system guide Designed for 6 months daily use	• VLU • Prevention of VLU recurrence	DNM	8	£96.97

MLB (n) multilayer bandage (number of layers), *SLB* single layer bandage, *AVW* adjustable Velcro wrap, *E* elastic, *SS* short stretch, *MLH (n)* multilayer hosiery (number of layers), *VLU* venous leg ulcer, *CO* chronic oedema, *DVT* deep venous thrombosis, *MAU* mixed aetiology ulcer, *DNM* does not mention

insufficiency is due to reflux or obstruction. The categories within CEAP are as follows:

- C0: No visible or palpable signs of venous disease.
- C1: Telangiectasias or reticular veins.
- C2: Varicose veins.
- C3: Oedema.
- C4: Changes in skin and subcutaneous tissue divided into two subclasses:
  - C4a Pigmentation or eczema
  - C4b Lipodermatosclerosis or atrophie blanche.
- C5: Healed venous ulcer
- C6: Active venous ulcer

Table 3.2 lists the British standards (BS 7505) for compression bandages, the corresponding USA classification, and the applicable CEAP indications for each standard.

It should be noted that consensus meetings in the field have challenged the notion of consigning a particular bandage type to one of the standards in Table 3.2, given the pressure exerted is dependent on the material and the tension applied [35]. One alternative way of categorising compression bandages is by their elasticity or stiffness. For example, bandages may be categorised depending on whether their maximal stretch at 10 N/cm bandage width is 0–10% (inelastic - rigid), 10–100% (inelastic - short stretch), or >100% (elastic - long stretch) [35]. Furthermore, compression bandages may either be single-layer, or multi-layered kits that comprise a

Table 3.2 British standard (BS 7505) and USA classifications for compression bandages, their pressure application, and suggested indications (adapted from [34])

British standard	USA Classification	Pressure applied (mmHg)	Suggested indication
3A	Light	<20	Mild C1–3; unable to apply/tolerate 3B.
3B	Class I (moderate)	21–30	Mild C1–3
3C	Class II (high)	31–40	Severe C2–3, C4 and higher, post thrombotic syndrome
3D	Class III (very high)	>40	C5–6 (if non-responsive to 3C, and if tolerated)

combination of elastic or inelastic bandages that are applied sequentially to provide additive benefits of different forms of compression.

3.5.1 Inelastic Compression Bandages

When characterising the effect of different compression bandages on patients, the static standing index (SSI) can be used to provide a measure of the difference in pressure applied when a patient moves from the supine to the standing position [36]. When compared to elastic bandages, inelastic bandages have a greater ability to provide a resistance to the outward force generated as muscles contract while a patient moves from a supine to standing position, or during activity. As such, the SSI is much greater for inelastic bandages than elastic bandages. Studies have shown that the increase in SSI for inelastic bandages also correlates with an increase in ejection fraction in patients with venous insufficiency, when compared to those wearing elastic compression bandages [37], thus improving the potential for VLU healing. Indeed, this has been highlighted in a recent study that conclusively demonstrated the benefit of inelastic compression therapy over elastic compression therapy in the treatment of VLUs [38]. A potential limitation of inelastic bandaging is the inability to conform to changes in leg volume as oedema increases (e.g. during standing) or decreases (e.g. at elevation during rest). As such, there can be a loss of pressure over time, which inevitably reduces the therapeutic benefit of the bandage and necessitates bandage replacement.

3.5.2 Elastic Compression Bandages

Due to the way that elastic compression bandages conform to changes in leg size, these bandages can sustain higher levels of compression than inelastic bandages during both activity and at rest. However, one potential limitation of this sustained pressure is the inability of patients to achieve respite from the compression when trying to achieve higher levels of standing pressure [37]. For this reason, elastic compression bandages are often included as part of a multi-layered bandage system, which may include inner absorbent layers for capturing excess exudate, or outer adhesive layers for holding the compression therapy in place and preventing slippage [39]. Emerging technologies have even shown the ability to convert an elastic bandage to an inelastic compression therapy simply via the attachment of non-stretchable patches to the outside of an elastic bandage once applied to a patient's leg [40].

3.6 Compression Hosiery

Compression hosiery in the form of stockings and other tubular garments can be used as an alternative to compression bandages, to apply a gradient of pressure across the length of the limb. The greatest pressure is generally applied distally at the ankle and reduced proximally towards the knee and thigh. While there has been some recent debate as to whether graduated pressure should be "progressive" (calf > ankle) [41], the general standard of care in UK and Ireland is "degressive" (ankle > calf). The inherent mechanical properties of compression hosiery, and indeed compression bandages, such as stiffness, elasticity, and elastic hysteresis, can be controlled by the type of materials and fabrication techniques utilised to form different microstructures during the manufacturing process [27].

Much the same as the British standards for compression bandages, the UK and Ireland generally have three classes of compression hosiery, which are related to the strength of compression applied; Class 1: light support; Class 2: medium support; Class 3: strong support. There are different varieties of compression hosiery for different body parts (e.g. below the knee stockings, thigh length stockings, socks, tights) and the sizes of these garments may be standard or made to measure. In addition to selecting the correct class and type of hosiery for the indication, it's important to correctly measure and fit compression hosiery, as well as providing the patient with clear instructions of use, in order to ensure comfort and improve compliance.

While compression hosiery can provide an effective alternative to compression bandages, there are several challenges with their use, primarily related to their application. It is important to consider the condition of the skin before prescribing compression hosiery as the application of hosiery may cause wounds in patients with fragile skin. Application of hosiery can be quite challenging for patients who have poor manual dexterity, particularly if the patient is frail and the required compression levels are high. Often a healthcare provider is required for assistance if the hosiery is Class 2 or 3, however zippers, Velcro systems, and specialised donning devices can help in hosiery application, albeit at an additional cost. For below the knee stockings, it is important to ensure they are not pulled up to the popliteal fossa as this location can result in stricture, skin irritation, or discomfort. Conversely, thigh-high stockings must be pulled high enough that they don't wrinkle when the knee is bent, which can then provide similar problems in the popliteal space. Finally, the difficulty in application of compression hosiery in patients with an active ulcer can also make for a painful process, although once applied, compression hosiery has been shown to reduce pain and aching in patients with symptomatic varicose veins [42].

3.7 Adjustable Velcro Wraps

A relatively new form of compression therapy that was the focus of a recent National Institute for Health and Care Excellence (NICE) medtech innovation briefing (MIB) [43] is the adjustable Velcro wrap (AVW). The features of these AVWs include an ability to provide:

- High pressure [44] (due to high wall stability [45])
- Comfort (due to breathability [46])
- Cost-effectiveness [43] (due to durability)
- Tolerance at rest (due to reduced stretch [47])
- Pleasing aesthetics (due to reduced bulkiness and an ability to conform to patients' shoes [48])
- An ability to allow patient autonomy in better managing the continuous application of therapeutic compression [44] (due to the ease of adjustability).

Traditionally, AVW systems have been used in the treatment of oedema [47] and lympoedema [44], however the limited clinical data for their use in treating VLUs has suggested that they may provide improvements in pain and depression, skin integrity, and self-care when compared to traditional compression bandages [49]. Furthermore, despite the significantly higher initial cost of AVWs compared to traditional compression bandages, these products have a 6-month minimum life-span and case studies have suggested that there are significant savings in expenditure over the course of compressive therapy. This is due to a reduction in healthcare provider time (due to the reduced frequency and length of home or clinic visits facilitated by easier self-management using AVWs), as well as a reduced amount of clinical waste [43]. Another potential benefit of AVWs over standard bandages is the ability to better sustain therapeutic levels of sub-bandage pressure over the course of treatment. Standard bandages are known to drastically reduce in pressure as swelling subsides, some by as much as 50% in 3 days [50], potentially depriving the patient of effectual treatment until seen again by a healthcare provider. AVWs allow for the adjustment and reapplication of lost pressure by the patient or care provider [44, 47].

One caveat to the use of AVWs in the treatment of chronic wounds is the need for identifying appropriate patient profiles for the various forms of these devices, based on the functionality of patients [51]. In general, the use of AVWs in the treatment of chronic wounds has demonstrated good potential to improve healing outcomes, quality of life, and healthcare costs when compared to traditional compression bandages or hosiery. However, evidence thus far is largely confined to case studies and small patient series, which are often reported in non-peer reviewed conference posters, so more robust clinical trials are needed to verify these preliminary findings [49].

3.8 General Limitations of Compression Therapy

3.8.1 Recording ABPI

Prior to the application of compression therapy the recording of Ankle to Bracial Pressure Index (ABPI) is recommended. This should be completed by professionals competent in such procedural issues and able to integrate the results with overall clinical assessment [3]. In 2017 the European Wound Management Association (EWMA) published an overview of clinical practice guidelines for the management of venous leg ulceration. An area of uncertainty was at what ABPI can compression be applied in the absence of specialist vascular assessment? As most VLU treatment practices and compression therapy applications are made by nurses, often working solo and in patients' homes, the need for guidelines to assist and inform practice and decision making is crucial. This document has highlighted that while the need for compression is well supported through ten international guidelines, the threshold at which one can apply compression and when a patient should be referred is less clear.

A further review of twenty clinical practice guidelines, consensus statements and position documents followed by consensus meetings identified contraindications for compression therapy and potential adverse events [52] and concluded that absolute and relative contraindications for compression are arterial occlusive disease and pulmonary oedema from congestive heart failure. They also recommend the ABPI as a standard assessment to determine sufficient arterial circulation. An ABPI $\leq$0.8–0.6 indicated significant arterial disease and use modified compression with caution and refer to a specialist. ABPI $<$0.5 indicative of critical ischemia and should not be compressed and referred to a vascular specialist. They do acknowledge that guidelines are conflicting in relation to ABPI but also caution that reliance on a single value as a cut-off point for treatment has been debated as it neither defines the transition between venous and arterial ulceration nor takes into account differences in perfusion pressure between the three vessels at the ankle. Reliance on a single ratio also fails to take into consideration other factors that may be important when defining the level of compression to apply including; limb shape; presence of bony prominences; skin condition; variability within the pressure measurement between three ankle pulses; the presence of other diseases such as diabetes or rheumatoid arthritis, and the patient's tolerance of compression [52].

3.9 Pressure Application

It has been suggested previously that the failings of compression therapy are likely to be more related to poor knowledge and application techniques of care providers than inherent failings of the products used [53]. Despite the application of pressure being core to the mechanism of compression therapy [54], and the desire for consistent, evidence-based treatments of VLUs [3], the application of standardised pressure is rarely achieved in clinical practice. For example, in a study of 891 healthcare providers, less than 10% were able to achieve a specified pressure of 50–60 mmHg upon applying a short-stretch compression bandage [55], while others have shown that professional experience has no bearing on adequate application of pressure [56]. This uncertainty in the application of correct pressure is a serious limitation in the current provision of treatment for several reasons. Firstly, there is strong evidence to suggest that a higher compression (e.g. >40 mmHg) is more effective than a low compression pressure (e.g. ≤20 mmHg) in promoting ulcer healing [3, 57], so incorrect pressure may be ineffectual. Secondly, mixed aetiology, arteriovenous ulcers occur in 15–30% of ulcer patients [7–9], and when the ABPI is moderate (0.5 > ABPI ≤ 0.85) compression should only be applied cautiously to maintain circulation [2, 30], so incorrect pressure may be dangerous. Finally, proper investigation of conflicting reports on the optimal form of compression therapy is hampered by the inability to reliably assess the provision of treatment in the context of chronic wound healing. For example, debate as to whether graduated pressure should be "degressive" (ankle > calf, as with traditional compression therapy) or "progressive" (calf > ankle) is invalid if the treatment provided is unknown [41]. Taken together, these points suggest that delays or failures in VLU healing may be attributed to an inability to accurately assess and consistently deliver compression therapy at pressure levels that are clinically proven.

While issues related to an inability to consistently deliver appropriate levels of sub-bandage pressure may be addressed through training, studies have shown the benefits of training to be temporary [58], so continued retraining is required. Other solutions to the provision of correct and consistent sub-bandage pressure may include the development of sensor technologies that offer the ability to provide feedback on the pressure applied. While a number of pressure sensing technologies currently exist, as yet, none of these fit the ideal criteria for routine clinical use [59], often due to cost, accuracy, or practical considerations. Ultimately the ability of patients to sense the correct level of pressure after being trained may prove the best means of ensuring consistency, especially when empowered to self-adjust their own compression therapy [60].

3.10 Non-compliance

Notwithstanding the consensus that compression is of benefit to VLU healing, it is not without its challenges for patients and impacts of their daily lives. Bandages are bulky and limit choices in foot wear. They can also be warm, which is particularly problematic in some climates, as treatment typically lasts 3–6 months and the 'treatment' time can be protracted. The outer layer often does not slide easily in bed clothes, consequently disturbing sleep, and their high visibility can act like a signal to others that the individual has a leg ulcer. Bandages have no colour choice so for those with darker skin their visibility is even greater. It is not surprising therefore that patient's can find it difficult to adhere to compression regimes.

Patient non-compliance ranges from 2% to 42% of patients in RCTs, or 9.7–80% in community studies [61]. Furthermore, compliance can have a dramatic impact on the healing rate of VLUs, with one previous study reporting a 78% healing rate in compliant patients versus 29% in non-compliant patients after 6 months [62]. The basis for non-compliance is complex and patient-specific. Proposed methods to address these issues include improving doctor-patient communication, pragmatic and progressive approaches of treatment that tailor to patient objections (e.g. pain will decrease with healing but should not be disregarded), forwarding patient and clinical education, and promoting patient empowerment [25, 62].

A systematic review by Weller et al. [63] to identify interventions for helping people adhere to compression treatments identified three RCTs [63–65]. Of these one did not return results applicable to the outcomes of the review and thus only two studies were identified. Meta-analysis was not possible due to different time point outcome evaluation and interventions.

In the review, one RCT among 67 participants compared a community-based socialisation and peer-support clinical (Leg Club) to home-based wound care [64]. At 3 months healing outcomes were 43% (12/28) versus 25% (7/28) respectively, relative risk (RR) 1.71 (95% confidence interval (CI) 0.79–3.71). At 6 months this increased to 45% (15/33) versus 29% (10/34) RR 1.55, (95% CI 0.81–2.93). The second RCT among 184 participants, compared a community-based exercise and behaviour modification clinic (Lively Legs) plus usual care compared with usual care [65]. At 18 months it was uncertain if there was a difference in the number of people healed with 55% (51/92) healed in Lively legs versus 45% (41/92) usual care RR 1.24, (95 % CI 0.93–1.67) due to possible imprecision around the result and risk of selection bias.

Most striking in the studies included in the latter review [63] was the low healing rates at three and 6 months. In the study by Edwards et al. [64], 43% versus 25% healed at 3 months and 45% versus 29% at 6 months, at both time points falling far short of an expected 50% healing rate at 3 months. In the study by Heinen et al. [65], 55% versus 44% healed at 18 months with a recurrence rate of 46% versus 56%. The review authors state their ability to draw firm conclusion is limited by the quality and number of trials and that at present it is not possible either to recommend or discourage educational interventions or nurse-led clinics care interventions over standard care in terms of increasing adherence to compression bandaging [63].

3.10.1 Evidence for Compression

A Cochrane systematic review [1] of compression for VLU has concluded from 48 RCTs reporting 59 comparisons among 4321 participants that compression increases ulcer healing rates compared with no compression; that multicomponent systems are more effective that single component systems, and that patients receiving 4LB heal faster than those allocated to SSB. A recent meta-analysis focusing only on 4LB versus SSB shows slightly different results than the Cochrane Review [66]. The latter review included seven RCTs among 1435 patients. At 12 or 16 weeks 51% (n = 259) ulcers healed completely in 4LB versus 46% (n = 234) in the SSB (RR 1.07 [95% CI 0.91–1.27] P = 0.41). However, a distinct difference is that O'Meara used individual patient data compared to De Cavello who used ulcer as the unit of analysis. Nonetheless, outcomes while superior were only slightly so.

The latter two reviews again highlight the limitations of healing outcomes when compression alone is considered. In the latter review, healing times were 73.6 ± 14.64 days and 83.8 ± 24.89 in 4LB and SSB respectively. The Cochrane review reported days to healing as 90 days versus 99 days respectively but again this is patient data and not ulcer data. Given the consensus that compression is the 'gold standard' it really falls short as after 12 weeks of treatment one can only expect an average of 44% in 4LB and 37% in SBB to heal and by 24 weeks this rises to 62% versus 61%. As compression therapy is a continuous treatment across 24 h a day, 7 days per week such outcomes are poor and do not constitute any significant advance in improved patient outcomes since the first studies.

3.11 Controversies in Compression

An observation from a study by Guest et al. 2013 raises an interesting topic for debate, in which healing outcomes in those not receiving compression was greater at 6 months follow-up than those in compression [67]. The study analysed patients on the GP registry in the United Kingdom on The Health Improvement Network (THIN) database. This database has been assessed as being representative of the UK population in terms of age, gender, and disease status. The study analysed data from three patient cohorts. The first two were drawn from the THIN database and the third from the results of an RCT completed in 2005/2006. Group 1 represented a random selection of 414 patients with VLU >3 months with high levels of wound exudate of which 20% (n = 74) never received compression and were compared with 74 who did. Cohort number two were drawn from the same database and included 255 patients with VLU>3 months in receipt of a skin protectant. Of these 66% (n = 164) never received compression and were compared with 164 who did. The third group were drawn from a previous RCT and included 23% (n = 19) who never received compression and matched with 19 who did. Across all three cohorts there were no significant differences between those receiving and not receiving compression based on patient characteristics, wound characteristics or co-morbidities. When all three cohorts were analysed for healing outcomes, significantly more patients healed at 6 months in the no compression group than the compression group ($P < 0.02$) although time to healing was not significantly different.

Guest et al. [67] have acknowledged the limitation of their analysis but notwithstanding this, some significant factors are highlighted. The first two cohorts represent normal routine clinical practice and thus 20% of patients are not in receipt of compression but the reasons for this are not determined. Healing outcomes in the first cohort are high at 47% versus 68% in compression versus no compression and are thus more in line with other studies of outcomes at 6 months. But, in the other two studies outcomes are far less favourable being as low as 6% in those receiving compression to the highest of 26% in those not receiving compression and included in the RCT. The authors do acknowledge that data collection was for the purpose of routine clinical care and not for research purpose but it serves to highlight the need for databases that can be used for research purposes. In a follow up commentary in the same journal, Partsch [68] reiterates that compression should be continued as the mainstay for treatment of venous leg ulceration and asserts that in most cases non-healing are due to inadequate care, mainly because of poor compression. He further argues that we need compression as we simply cannot escape from gravity but that there is a need for better knowledge of effective forms of compression to counteract gravity and better skills in bandaging techniques [68].

While RCTs are considered the 'gold standard' to assess the efficacy of interventions, they are not without their limitation in wound healing studies. Gethin et al. [69] reported on 102 RCTs in VLU and identified 79 different study outcomes, of which healing was the most frequent ($n = 34$) with only 40 trials reporting a definition of healing. A significant limitation as highlighted in this review was that only five studies made reference to the validity and reliability of methods used to assess the wound and of these only one reported on measures of validity. A second important finding is the small study size with mean trial size being 108 and a median of 83, potentially limiting generalizability. An important finding as only 20% of wound care trials are sufficiently large enough to show a statistically significant treatment effect, should one exist [70].

3.12 Conclusion

Compression therapy is not new. It is regarded as the first line treatment for uncomplicated VLU. Yet, it remains fraught with difficulties. The IRR of the application technique using bandages is rarely evaluated and when it is, it is poor, bandages are unsightly and patients struggle to cope with them, healing outcomes after 6 months of therapy leave significant scope for improvement, compression is expensive and costly for the individual and the health service. The need for better and alternative systems is well acknowledge and future research must focus on the characteristics of those who heal compared to those who do not heal. RCTs should have standardised reporting times and consistent terminology, and research into adjunct therapies to augment compression therapy is required.

References

1. O'Meara SM, Cullum N, Nelson EA, Dumville J. Compression for venous leg ulcers. Cochrane Database Syst Rev. 2012;11:CD000265. https://doi.org/10.1002/14651858.CD000265.pub3.
2. Ratliff CR, Yates S, McNichol L, Gray M. Compression for primary prevention, treatment, and prevention of recurrence of venous leg ulcers: an evidence-and consensus-based algorithm for care across the continuum. J Wound Ostomy Continence Nurs. 2016;43(4):347.

3. Franks P, Barker J, Collier M, Gethin G, Haesler E, Jawien A, et al. Management of patients with venous leg ulcers: challenges and current best practice. J Wound Care. 2016; 25:S1.
4. Guest JF, Ayoub N, McIlwraith T, Uchegbu I, Gerrish A, Weidlich D, et al. Health economic burden that wounds impose on the National Health Service in the UK. BMJ Open. 2015;5(12):e009283.
5. de Carvalho MR, de Andrade IS, de Abreu AM, Ribeiro APL, Peixoto BU, de Oliveira BGRB. All about compression: a literature review. J Vasc Nurs. 2016;34(2): 47–53.
6. Reeder S, Maessen-Visch M, Langendoen S, de Roos K, Neumann H. The recalcitrant venous leg ulcer–a never ending story? Phlebologie. 2013;42(6):332–9.
7. Woo KY, Sears K. Knowledge, attitude, and practice in the management of mixed arteriovenous leg ulcers. Int J Low Extrem Wounds. 2016;15(1):52–7.
8. Humphreys ML, Stewart AHR, Gohel MS, Taylor M, Whyman MR, Poskitt KR. Management of mixed arterial and venous leg ulcers. Br J Surg. 2007;94(9):1104–7.
9. Ghauri ASK, Nyamekye I, Grabs AJ, Farndon JR, Poskitt KR. The diagnosis and management of mixed arterial/venous leg ulcers in community-based clinics. Eur J Vasc Endovasc Surg. 1998;16(4):350–5.
10. Marin JA, Woo KY. Clinical characteristics of mixed arteriovenous leg ulcers: a descriptive study. J Wound Ostomy Cont Nurs. 2017;44(1):41–7.
11. Haesler E. Evidence summary: managing lymphoedema: compression therapy. Wound Pract Res J Aust Wound Manag Assoc. 2016;24(4):233.
12. AnitaHobday. Use of compression therapy in patients with lymphoedema. Nurs Stand. 2016;30(27):50–60.
13. Cooper G, Bagnall A. Prevalence of lymphoedema in the UK: focus on the southwest and West Midlands. Br J Community Nurs. 2016;21(Sup4):S6–S14.
14. Moffatt CJ, Keeley V, Franks PJ, Rich A, Pinnington LL. Chronic oedema: a prevalent health care problem for UK health services. Int Wound J. 2017;14(5):772–81.
15. Vlajinac H, Marinkovic J, Maksimovic M, Radak D. Factors related to venous ulceration: a cross-sectional study. Angiology. 2014;65(9):824–30.
16. Heinen MM, Persoon A, van de Kerkhof P, Otero M, van Achterberg T. Ulcer-related problems and health care needs in patients with venous leg ulceration: a descriptive, cross-sectional study. Int J Nurs Stud. 2007;44(8):1296–303.
17. Apollonio A, Antignani PL, Di Salvo M, Failla G, Guarnera G, Mosti G, et al. A large Italian observational multicentre study on vascular ulcers of the lower limbs (Studio Ulcere Vascolari). Int Wound J. 2016;13(1):27–34.
18. Price P, Harding K. Measuring health related quality of life in patients with chronic leg ulcers. Wounds. 1996;8:91–4.
19. Rich A, McLachlan L. How living with a leg ulcer affects people's daily life: a nurse-led study. J Wound Care. 2003;12(2):51–4.
20. Hopman WM, Vandenkerkhof EG, Carley ME, Harrison MB. Health-related quality of life at healing in individuals with chronic venous or mixed-venous leg ulceration: a longitudinal assessment. J Adv Nurs. 2016;72(11):2869–78.
21. Posnett J, BA D, Gottrup F, MD D, MSc HL, Saal G, BA M. The resource impact of wounds on health-care providers in Europe. J Wound Care. 2009;18(4):154.
22. Guest JF, Fuller GW, Vowden P. Venous leg ulcer management in clinical practice in the UK: costs and outcomes. Int Wound J. 2018;15(1):29–37.
23. Harrison MB, VanDenKerkhof EG, Hopman WM, Graham ID, Carley ME, Nelson EA. The Canadian Bandaging Trial: Evidence-informed leg ulcer care and the effectiveness of two compression technologies. BMC Nurs. 2011;10:20.
24. Scriven JM, Taylor LE, Wood AJ, Bell PR, Naylor AR, London NJ. A prospective randomised trial of four-layer versus short stretch compression bandages for the treatment of venous leg ulcers. Ann R Coll Surg Engl. 1998;80(3):215–20.
25. Harding K. Challenging passivity in venous leg ulcer care – the ABC model of management. Int Wound J. 2016;13(6):1378–84.

26. Rockson SG. Intermittent pneumatic compression therapy. In: Lee B-B, Rockson SG, Bergan J, editors. Lymphedema: a concise compendium of theory and practice. Cham: Springer International Publishing; 2018. p. 443–8.
27. Liu R, Guo X, Lao TT, Little T. A critical review on compression textiles for compression therapy: textile-based compression interventions for chronic venous insufficiency. Text Res J. 2017;87(9):1121–41.
28. Thomas S. The production and measurement of sub-bandage pressure: Laplace's Law revisited. J Wound Care. 2014;23(5):234–46.
29. Mosti G. Compression in mixed ulcers. Veins and Lymphatics, [S.l.], June 2016. ISSN 2279-7483. https://doi.org/10.4081/vl.2016.5986. Accessed 10 Oct 2018.
30. Mosti G, Iabichella ML, Partsch H. Compression therapy in mixed ulcers increases venous output and arterial perfusion. J Vasc Surg. 2012;55(1):122–8.
31. Mosti G, Cavezzi A, Massimetti G, Partsch H. Recalcitrant venous leg ulcers may heal by outpatient treatment of venous disease even in the presence of concomitant arterial occlusive disease. Eur J Vasc Endovasc Surg. 2016;52(3):385–91.
32. Eklöf B, Rutherford RB, Bergan JJ, Carpentier PH, Gloviczki P, Kistner RL, et al. Revision of the CEAP classification for chronic venous disorders: consensus statement. J Vasc Surg. 2004;40(6):1248–52.
33. Beebe HG, Bergan JJ, Bergqvist D, Eklof B, Eriksson I, Goldman MP, et al. Classification and grading of chronic venous disease in the lower limbs. a consensus statement. Eur J Vasc Endovasc Surg. 1996;12(4):487–92.
34. Attaran RR, Ochoa Chaar CI. Compression therapy for venous disease. Phlebology. 2016;32(2):81–8.
35. Partsch H, Clark M, Mosti G, Steinlechner E, Schuren JAN, Abel M, et al. Classification of compression bandages: practical aspects. Dermatol Surg. 2008;34(5):600–9.
36. Partsch H. The static stiffness index: a simple method to assess the elastic property of compression material in vivo. Dermatol Surg. 2006;31(6):625–30.
37. Mosti G, Mattaliano V, Partsch H. Inelastic compression increases venous ejection fraction more than elastic bandages in patients with superficial venous reflux. Phlebology. 2008;23(6):287–94.
38. Mosti G. Venous ulcer treatment requires inelastic compression. Phlebologie. 2018;47(01):7–12.
39. Armstrong DG, Meyr A. Compression therapy for the treatment of chronic venous insufficiency. U: UpToDate, Mills JL, Eidt JF ur UpToDate [Internet]. 2017.
40. Mosti G, Partsch H. A new two component compression system turning an elastic bandage into an inelastic compression device: interface pressure, stiffness, and haemodynamic effectiveness. Eur J Vasc Endovasc Surg. 2018;55(1):126–31.
41. Mosti G. Progressive or degressive compression pressure profile in patients with chronic venous disorders of the lower limb. Veins Lymphatics. 2014;3(1). https://doi.org/10.4081/vl.2014.2235
42. Kakkos SK, Timpilis M, Patrinos P, Nikolakopoulos KM, Papageorgopoulou CP, Kouri AK, et al. Acute effects of graduated elastic compression stockings in patients with symptomatic varicose veins: a randomised double blind placebo controlled trial. Eur J Vasc Endovasc Surg. 2018;55(1):118–25.
43. NICE. The Juxta-CURES adjustable compression system for treating venous leg ulcers. Available from: https://www.nice.org.uk/advice/mib25.
44. Damstra RJ, Partsch H. Prospective, randomized, controlled trial comparing the effectiveness of adjustable compression Velcro wraps versus inelastic multicomponent compression bandages in the initial treatment of leg lymphedema. J Vasc Surg Venous Lymphatic Disord. 2013;1(1):13–9.
45. Dissemond J, Assenheimer B, Bültemann A, Gerber V, Gretener S, Kohler-von Siebenthal E, et al. Compression therapy in patients with venous leg ulcers. J Dtsch Dermatol Ges. 2016;14(11):1072–87.
46. Appel J. Compression wrap and garment. Google Patents; 2007.
47. Mosti G, Cavezzi A, Partsch H, Urso S, Campana F. Adjustable Velcro® compression devices are more effective than inelastic bandages in reducing venous edema in the initial treatment phase: a randomized controlled trial. Eur J Vasc Endovasc Surg. 2015;50(3):368–74.

48. Williams AF. A review of the evidence for adjustable compression wrap devices. J Wound Care. 2016;25(5):242–7.
49. Williams A. An updated review of the evidence for adjustable compression wrap devices in the lower limb. Nurse Prescr. 2017;15(Sup10):6–13.
50. Protz K, Heyer K, Verheyen-Cronau I, Augustin M. Loss of interface pressure in various compression bandage systems over seven days. Dermatology. 2014;229(4):343–52.
51. Ehmann S, Bock K. Case report to demonstrate the need for selection criteria for optimal adjustable Velcro wrap prescription. J Wound Care. 2018;27(Sup1):S10–S7.
52. Andriessen A, Apelqvist J, Mosti G, Partsch H, Gonska C, Abel M. Compression therapy for venous leg ulcers: risk factors for adverse events and complications, contraindications - a review of present guidelines. Eur J Dermatol Venereol. 2017. https://doi.org/10.1111/jdv.14390. [Epub ahead of print].
53. Partsch H, Mortimer P. Compression for leg wounds. Br J Dermatol. 2015;173(2):359–69.
54. Hague A, Pherwani A, Rajagopalan S. Role of compression therapy in pathophysiology of the venous system in lower limbs. Surgeon. 2017;15(1):40–6.
55. Protz K, Heyer K, Dörler M, Stücker M, Hampel-Kalthoff C, Augustin M. Compression therapy: scientific background and practical applications. J Dtsch Dermatol Ges. 2014;12(9): 794–801.
56. Zarchi K, Jemec GE. Delivery of compression therapy for venous leg ulcers. JAMA Dermatol. 2014;150(7):730–6.
57. Milic DJ, Zivic SS, Bogdanovic DC, Jovanovic MM, Jankovic RJ, Milosevic ZD, et al. The influence of different sub-bandage pressure values on venous leg ulcers healing when treated with compression therapy. J Vasc Surg. 2010;51(3):655–61.
58. Tidhar D, Keren E, Brandin G, Yogev M, Armer JM. Effectiveness of compression bandaging education for wound care nurses. J Wound Care. 2017;26(11):625–31.
59. Partsch H, Clark M, Bassez S, Benigni J-P, Becker F, Blazek V, et al. Measurement of lower leg compression in vivo: recommendations for the performance of measurements of interface pressure and stiffness. Dermatol Surg. 2006;32(2):224–33.
60. Mosti G, Partsch H. Self-management by firm, non-elastic adjustable compression wrap device [Translation of Druckmessungen unter Klettverschluss-Kompression-Selbstbehandlung durch feste, unelastische Beinwickelung]. Veins Lymphatics. 2017;6(3):88–90.
61. Moffatt C, Kommala D, Dourdin N, Choe Y. Venous leg ulcers: patient concordance with compression therapy and its impact on healing and prevention of recurrence. Int Wound J. 2009;6(5):386–93.
62. Rustempašić N. Causes and consequences of patient noncompliance to compression therapy of leg venous ulcers. Folia Med Fac Med Univ Saraeviensis. 2012;47(1):14–20.
63. Weller CD, Buchbinder R, Johnston RV. Interventions for helping people adhere to compression treatments for venous leg ulceration. Cochrane Database Syst Rev. 2016;3:CD008378.
64. Edwards H, Courtney M, Finlayson K, Shuter P, Lindsay E. A randomised controlled trial of a community nursing intervention: improved quality of life and healing for clients with chronic leg ulcers. J Clin Nurs. 2009;18(11):1541–9.
65. Heinen M, Borm G, van der Vleuten C, Evers A, Oostendorp R, van Acherberg T. The Lively Legs self-management programme increased physical activity and reduced wound days in leg ulcer patients: Results from a randomised controlled trial. Int J Nurs Stud. 2012;49(2):151–61.
66. De Carvalho MR, Peixoto BU, Silveira IA, Oliveria B. A meta-analysis to compare four-layer to short-stretch compression bandaging for venous leg ulcer healing. Ostomy Wound Manage. 2018;64(5):30–7.
67. Guest JF, Charles H, Cutting KF. Is it time to re-appraise the role of compression in non-healing venous leg ulcers? J Wound Care. 2013;22(9):453–60.
68. Partsch H. Commentary. J Wound Care. 2013;22(9):461.
69. Gethin G, Killeen F, Devane D. Heterogeneity of wound outcome measures in RCTs of treatments for VLUs: a systematic review. J Wound Care. 2015;24(5):211–2, 4, 6 passim.
70. Hodgson R, Allen R, Broderick E, Bland J, Dumville J, Ashby R, et al. Funding source and the quality of reports of chronic wounds trials: 2004 to 2011. Trials. 2014;15(1):19.

Chapter 4
Difficult to Compress Legs with Venous Disease

Mieke Flour

Abstract Patients suffering from venous disease may encounter situations which render compression treatment challenging at least temporarily while complications are managed.

Aside from the skin changes and/or ulceration itself, the leg can present anatomical or functional problems, like skin atrophy or impaired mobility, frank deformity or scarring. Motivation and ability to self-management are personal factors which play a role; other challenges may come from the patient's socio-cultural or economic situation. Even motivated people may become discouraged by working demands/circumstances or by climatological factors. Temporary or remaining concurrent medical problems may be diagnosed to be contra-indications for standard compression treatment. In regions where there is a paucity of skilled caregivers, instruction of the appliers or of the patient itself, and follow-up of treatment may be difficult to arrange. Availability of materials is not always evident in some countries or in some of their remote regions due to issues of marketing and infrastructure. The same holds for provision and organisation of care, rendering optimal compression therapy too exceptional and/or too expensive.

These challenges by themselves or in combination, are the main reason to making it difficult to compress legs with venous disease.

Keywords Compression treatment · Venous disease · Variations · Challenges · Adapted compression techniques · Combination of compression devices

4.1 Introduction

To treat a limb with venous insufficiency, whenever possible, the choice of compression should be guided by evidence or consensus.

Results of studies and ensuing guidelines cannot always be transferred to the clinical setting of everyday practice. One of the many reason for this is that the

---

M. Flour (✉)
Dermatology, University Hospitals Leuven, Leuven, Belgium

R. Mani et al. (eds.), *Compression and Chronic Wound Management*,
https://doi.org/10.1007/978-3-030-01195-6_4

baseline characteristics of the real-life population with venous insufficiency or with an open leg ulcer seem to be more complex than the included study population. Contra-indications and complications may defer or interdict compression treatment.

One must also consider the patient's condition in a holistic way (mobility, ability to care for him/herself), or the need for assistance in applying compression devices, the state of the wound (exudative, infected or clean granulating), the type and size of the bandage/stocking and the optimal frequency of its replacement [1].

The most frequently encountered challenges in daily practice of treating venous ulcers are skin problems or wound complications on the limb to be treated, extreme obesity, disproportionate anatomical contours or dysfunctional and disfigured limbs, and co-morbidities which result in medical contra-indications for compression treatment.

Other challenges may come from the patient's socio-cultural or economic situation or circumstances of living like climate, availability of care and of materials, and cultural beliefs. Some of these aspects may render standard compression treatment difficult to implement, and then the caregiver and the patient will have to adapt treatment to what is possible and practically feasible within the boundaries of their expertise and responsibilities.

4.2 The Patient's Clinical Situation

This title refers to the local (ulcer itself), regional (the limb) and systemic (general health) conditions.

Local skin conditions may form a temporary or relative contra-indication for some types of compression treatment.

Oozing dermatitis and diffuse maceration of the skin ask for frequent dressing changes or other management decisions which may interfere with stockings or sustained bandaging.

Acute infection of the limb must be cared for before focusing on compression devices: the pain, fragility of the inflamed and swollen or blistering skin in patients with erysipelas, and the need to closely monitor the progression of the clinical signs force us to postpone compression for some time, and to choose for leg elevation instead during these few first days.

Intolerance or hypersensitivity/allergy to one of the components of the dressings, bandages or stockings is another reason to interrupt compression until skin tests confirm and document the responsible allergen. Most often, contact allergy to compression devices is due to latex, adhesives, coloring agents or fabric finishing chemicals. Recent development of "medicated stockings" and the manufacturing of "smart or antiseptic fabrics" include a certain risk for developing contact allergy to the added ingredients.

Irritant or allergic dermatitis, and the fragile skin especially due to high age or prolonged usage of corticosteroids may not tolerate high pressure values or may be traumatized by the application of rough materials onto the non-protected skin at bony prominences or overlying the tendons and joints.

Some phlebological patients present with limbs that have a hard indurated or sclerotic ankle and gaiter area, with or without ulceration, and a swollen soft obese upper part (Fig. 4.1). The "champagne bottle" leg is a challenge for effective compression treatment especially in cases presenting with heavily obese thighs or arthrosis in the knee.

Due to limited mobility the skin may be oedematous, with papillomatous lesions due to lymph stasis, or presenting myxedematous changes like those seen in diabetes and thyroid disease. Secondary skin changes may be so prevalent that they mask the underlying venous insufficiency, documented by Duplex and imaging. The needs for mobilisation and compression of tissues is not always equal in different compartments of the leg, and many times compression treatment will have to be adapted towards a combination of different materials and techniques (Figs. 4.1 and 4.2).

The pathological changes in advanced stages of venous hypertension not only affect the skin but also the deeper subcutaneous tissues, the joints, tendons and in

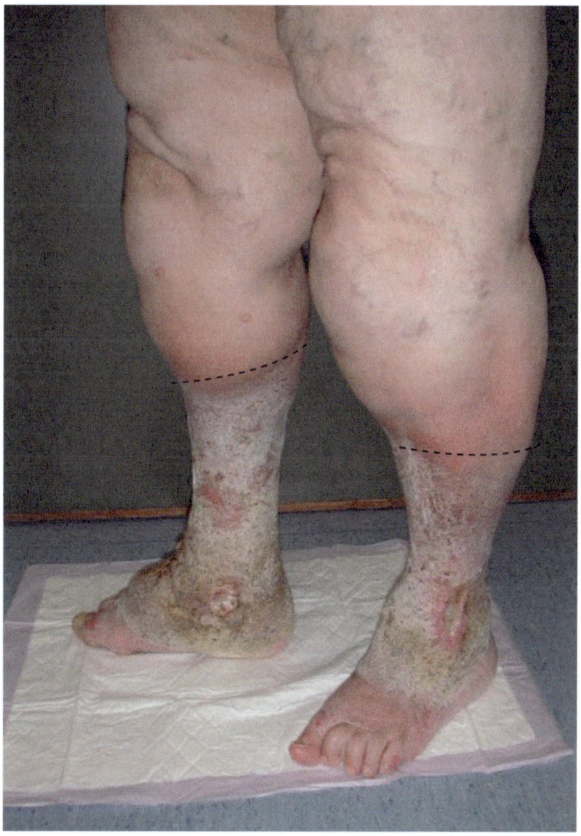

Fig. 4.1 Obese limbs may need to be divided into manageable parts which can be compressed using several different materials and methods

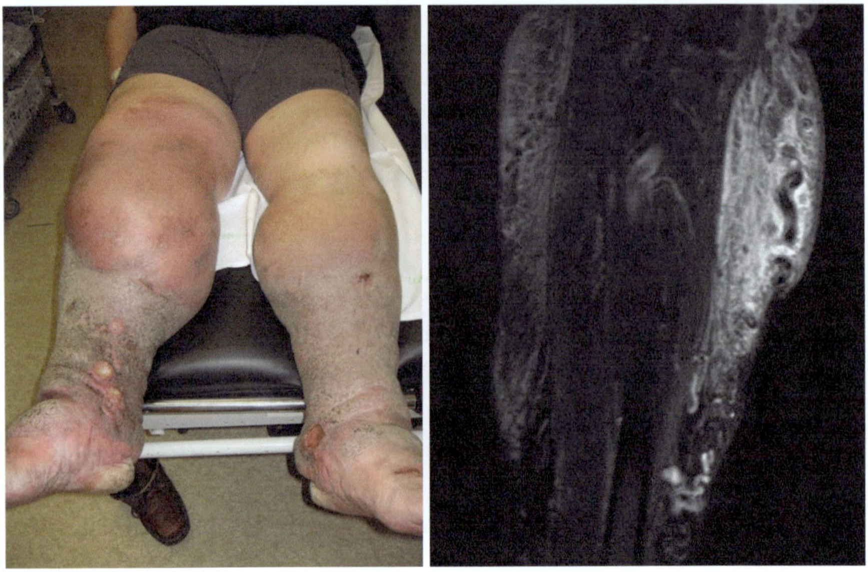

Fig. 4.2 Long term intake of corticosteroids resulted in skin atrophy in a transplant patient. A subcutaneous bag of accumulated lymph-like fluid separates the deep tissue planes

some cases even the bone. MRI and CT imaging reveals the thickened sclerotic alteration which can reach 0.5–2 cm deep. This may lead to an almost complete loss of ankle mobility and hence of calf muscle pump function and so exacerbate ambulatory venous hypertension. Fibrotic tissue will react differently to applied compression forces than would normal skin. We do not really know how tissue inflammation is influenced by mechanical forces, and how cellular metabolism will react to it.

The opposite extreme is represented in limbs where the skin is very thin and atrophic due to several reasons like long term corticosteroid medication for COPD, rheumatologic conditions or for preventing rejection of transplanted organs. In these conditions, the dermis has lost all elasticity and the ensuing venous and lymphatic drainage function, and passively gives way to the accumulation of tissue fluid (pooling by dependency) during the day (Fig. 4.3). Contention of oedema is needed although the skin is so fragile that mechanical trauma too easily results in wounding. Also, the fluid inside the compressed tissues may further separate layers of the atrophic subcutaneous tissue components (décollement). On imaging with MRI in two kidney transplant patients with a long survival and therefore long-time intake of corticosteroids, we found that this well delineated bag of accumulated lymph-like fluid was situated just outside the deep fascia, underneath the atrophic subcutis. Standard application of bandages had started to dissect the tissues layers further at both ends; so, the fluid had to be evacuated first to re-approximate the tissues. Compression treatment in these cases needs to combine maximal skin protection with sustained but adapted lower pressure.

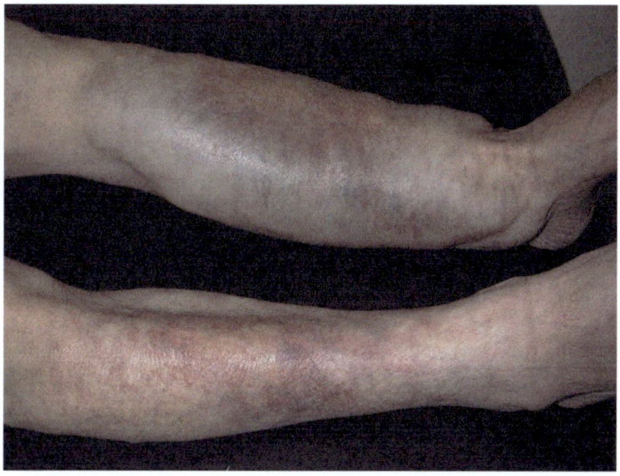

Fig. 4.3 Secondary skin changes in venous insufficiency may be so prevalent that they mask the underlying venous aetiology, documented by Duplex and imaging

Leg oedema or scarring disfigurement following trauma or surgery present a special challenge to adequate compression treatment. With the advancement of oncologic and reparative surgery, more limbs are saved that would have been amputated in previous decades. In reconstructive surgery, circumferential or degloving injuries may result in odd shapes of dysmorphic limbs, often presenting "entrapment" of venous and lymphatic drainage routes, loss of calf pump function, inhomogenous consistency of tissues with scarring and with areas where the skin is directly attached to the underlying bone or bulging muscle compartments that have no function in mobility and venous return due to interruption of tendons (Fig. 4.4). In these cases, the therapeutic goal is oedema reduction, support of functional mobility and restoring a nearly normal shape. Protective or draining padding must be carefully positioned to accommodate for uneven tissue characteristics and points of high pressure. The compressive system must not hinder revalidation exercises.

Systemic comorbidities may represent the major problem in patients with venous ulceration.

When we stand erect, the venous return from the foot to the heart is secured by a multi-organ pumping co-operation and requires a normal functioning of the heart, the peripheral arteries, the microcirculation, venous return and lymphatic drainage systems, muscle pump mechanisms, and normal pulmonary/thoracic biomechanics. Any one of these elements or a combination of factors can become defective, resulting in abnormal tissue circulation.

Patients suffering from a healed or active leg ulcer are usually elderly and sometimes in poor general health. Co-morbidities such as congestive heart failure, neuropathy and peripheral arterial disease present challenging situations. In endemic regions neuropathy due to diabetes or Hansen's disease or other infections must be considered, as well as sickle cell disease and tropical infections causing ulcerations or skin changes. Reduction of oedema must occur gradually to prevent cardio-pulmonary distress. Peripheral arteriopathy is not an absolute contraindication for compression therapy if we can adapt the technique and materials. Short stretch ban-

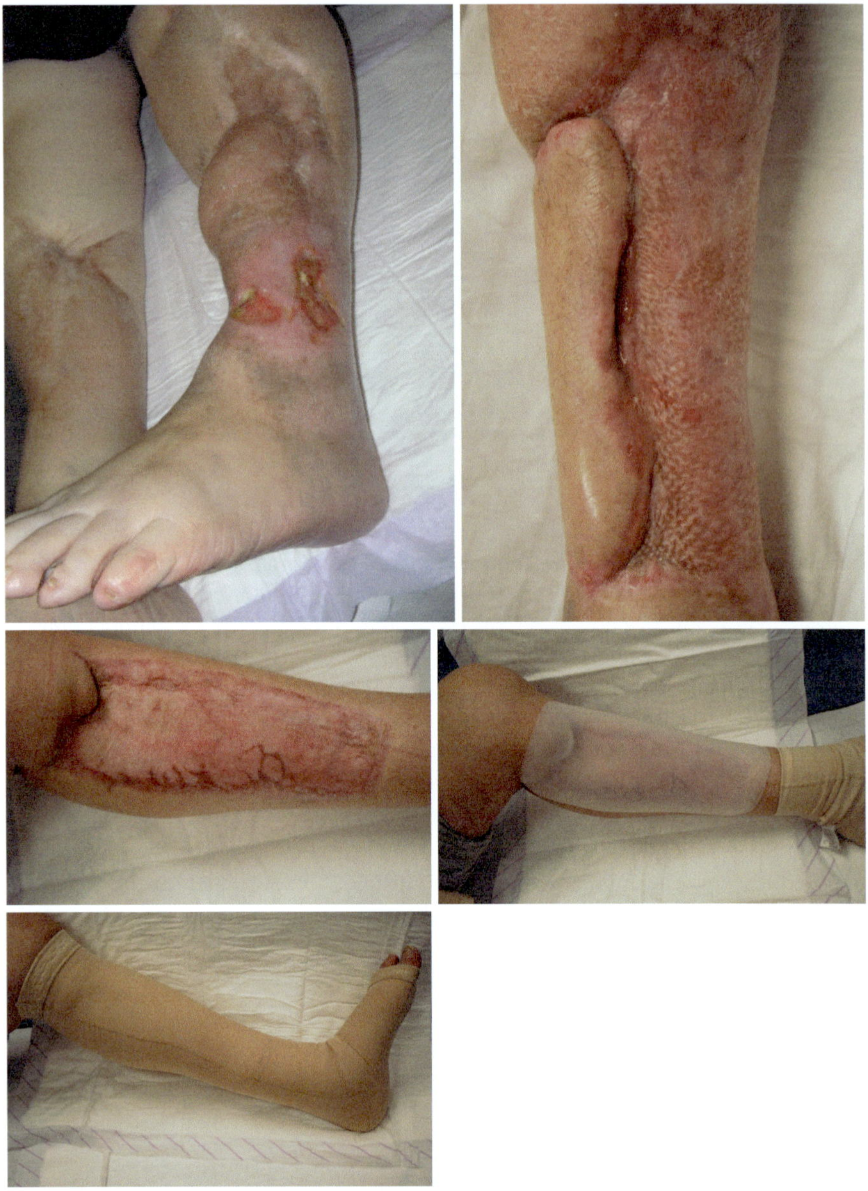

Fig. 4.4 Surgical reconstruction after major trauma may result in a scarred inhomogeneous or hemodynamically unfunctional limb. Prior to compression, correction or optimisation of the limb shape is necessary (e.g. here this was achieved using a silicone orthosis)

dages or any other compression system applied with a lowered resting pressure may be tolerated when peripheral systolic pressure is superior to 80 mmHg. It is standard procedure that assessment of the arterial status must precede any decision to apply compression treatment.

Since decades in many countries the prevalence of overweight and obesity has increased sharply for both adults and children. Being obese increases the risk of many diseases and health conditions, including hypertension, type 2 diabetes, coronary heart disease, osteoarthritis, sedentary lifestyle and loss of general condition [2]. These conditions represent challenges and potential contra-indications for compression treatment.

Neuropathy and micro-angiopathy due to diabetes and to hypertension are loco-regional medical conditions to be considered when prescribing compression treatment.

4.3 Adapting the Compression Techniques or Compression Materials and Devices to the Clinical Difficulties

When surgery is not an option or has only partial results, compression treatment is a valuable and effective choice. High compression levels and higher stiffness are more effective than low pressure by very elastic materials or bandaging systems. Protective padding is best used on sites of high pressure like prominent bone or tendon, and "fillers" will be added in places where compression is inadequate due to anatomical configuration: in the retro- and sub-malleolar region, where skin alterations and venous ulcers tend to occur. This is also referred to elsewhere in this book (see Chapter by Partsch and Mani).

The leg ulcer may need different wound management according to wound characteristics; the frequency of dressing changes will influence the choice of compression materials.

Local wound management should not be underestimated, nevertheless it has been shown that compression treatment is more important than topical wound management for venous ulcer healing.

When frequent dressing changes are required for an exuding ulcer, the wound needs to be readily accessible. Bandages or stockings are more appropriate in these cases than any type of sustained compression left in place for a longer period. In a later phase, healing, granulating ulcers can be treated with a dressing left in place for several days. In this situation, any type of compression may theoretically be chosen: Unna-boot, multi-layer/multicomponent or analogue systems, stockings in

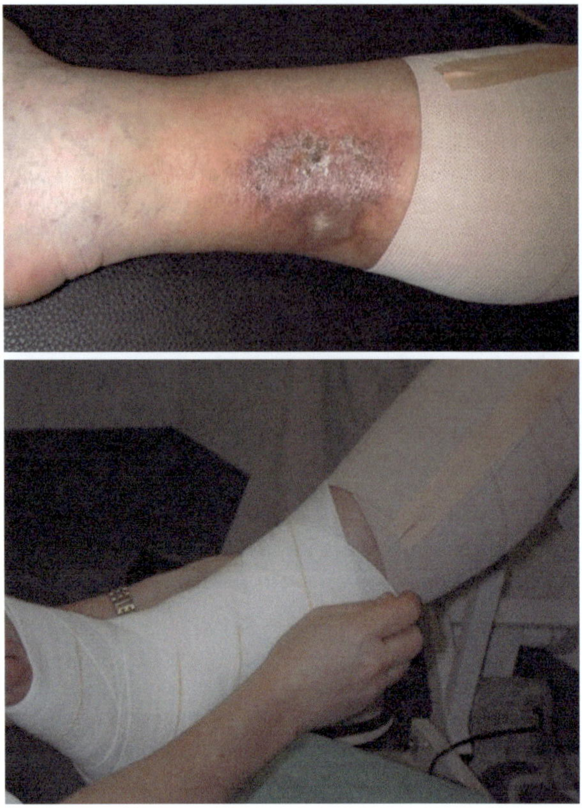

Fig. 4.5 Adapted compression treatment combining a sustained bandage left in place for several days at the calf level, and a multilayer stiff bandage at the distal part permitting daily wound treatment

single or in superposition. “Freshly” grafted leg ulcers need gentle care and thus dressings left in place for some days [3].

Heavily exuding or complicated wounds and oozing dermatitis in oedematous limbs are situations where sustained compression is technically difficult to realise. Daily application of topical preparations or dressings and clean bandages is more appropriate. In cases where this results in insufficient control of the swelling or if non-compliance to compression treatment will impair healing, one may consider sustained compression of only the calf if the skin in this area is healthy. An option is then to apply cohesive or adhesive bandages proximally, leaving the possibility to treat and to bandage the most distal part of the leg on a daily frequency (Fig. 4.5).

Intermittent pneumatic compression treatment will effectively complement treatment for these patients.

When there is edema or lipodermatosclerosis many authors will prefer treatment with a reasonable degree of stiffness. This will apply to the clinical stages C3 to C6 of the CEAP scoring and classification system of venous disorders [4].

In bedridden individuals a lighter compression will do, while for mobile persons the compression treatment needs to be more accurate and sustained.

Compression will be different for active mobile people compared to wheelchair-dependent patients or those with limited joint mobility of ankle, knee, hip and hands. In the latter, ankylosis impairs venous pump function, and the associated reduced muscle strength often makes it impossible to don or to take off the compression device without help/assistance. Joint symptoms are frequent in the elderly population presenting with venous ulceration. Superposition of low pressure stockings or sustained short stretch compression may be a good choice.

The pressure applied by a bandage or stocking is inversely proportional to the radius and may rise to high values on thin legs. The shape and consistency of the limb may cause problems just like the ankle circumference. The normal range of ankle diameter for compression devices, especially stockings, is between 18 and 25 cm.

Pressure values around 40 mmHg or more at the ankle are generally recommended to heal a venous leg ulcer. For reduction of edema, much less is needed since pressures as low as 6–20 mmHg may be effective. We do not know what mechanical forces are needed or how much is beneficial to impact on the indurated inflamed peri-ulcer skin.

Special situations require creative solutions: skin atrophy, heavily exuding wounds, heterogenous consistency of tissues, contact allergy, non-venous co-morbidities.

Deviation from recommended standards and guidelines may be dictated by the anatomy and function of the limb to treat. In addition, some situations ask for a combination of known standard techniques treating different parts of a leg in his separate most appropriate way. This may result in treating one part with a sustained bandaging technique, and the other part with bandages and dressings that are changed daily (Fig. 4.5). With experience and practice, care givers can adapt the compression therapy to the individual needs of the patient, reporting the reasons to do so, documenting treatment outcomes and considering the physical laws of compression treatment.

The pressure values indicated in the guidelines for compression treatment are deducted from investigations measuring the interface pressure, the tissue and the intra-luminal venous or lymphatic pressures and compression or occlusion of veins. In other words, pressures are prescribed based on the impact of compression upon the vessels. It is much more difficult to measure and to predict the effects on living pathological tissues as in lipodermatosclerosis. Ulcer healing in these indurated areas is substantially delayed. Mechanical forces influence the biological behaviour of the fibroblasts and other tissue cells, resulting in remodelling of structural molecules like collagen in fibrotic tissues. Very little is known about this aspect of compression treatment in vivo. There is no foundation for suggesting a specific amount of pressure to be applied to achieve clinical benefit in this field.

Nevertheless, clinical experience suggests that "massaging" of the tissues by short stretch stiff bandaging materials and application techniques results in softening of fibrotic areas even under low resting pressures, analogous to what is seen in the treatment of hypertrophic burn scars. Following efficient correction/optimisa-

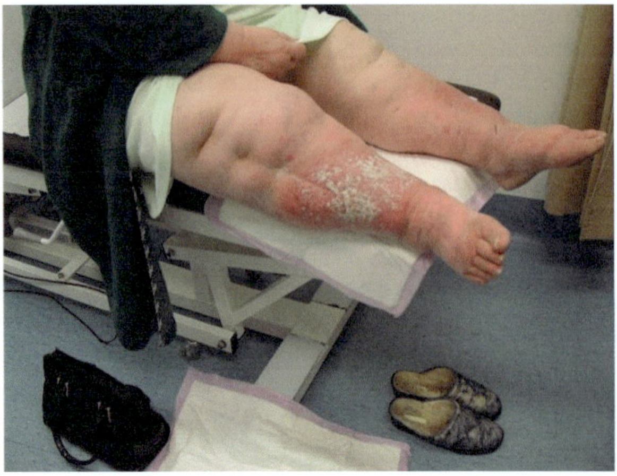

Fig. 4.6 Compression treatment shall be adapted to the ambitions and possibilities of care giver and patient alike. The major practical difficulty of compression treatment, and the best predicting factor for ulcer resistance or recurrence is "non-compliance" by the caregiver or the patient, for various reasons

tion of venous return with surgery and compression, a distinct and apparent reduction in fibrosis can be achieved, including a good restoration of function.

More attention is needed regarding compression in patients suffering from obesity and metabolic syndrome. Since losing weight will take many months and much effort, compression treatment needs to be adapted to the ambitions or possibilities of caregivers and patients alike (Fig. 4.6). This may call for lowering the pressure if bandages and stockings roll down, applying a layer purely to correct the shape of the leg, ordering stockings of a lesser compression class which are made to measure, and superposition of light stockings. If the patient can tolerate them, adhesive and cohesive bandages will stay in place much easier but choosing the most effective bandaging technique may be a major challenge even for experienced caregivers. The need for mobilisation and compression of tissues is not always equal in different compartments of the leg, and many times compression treatment will have to be adapted towards a combination of different materials and techniques. Obese limbs may need to be divided in manageable parts which can be compressed by several different materials and methods, not necessarily the same for the whole limb (Fig. 4.1).

When there is severe disfigurement of the leg or overweight patients may find it difficult to self-apply or readjust the so-called adjustable compression systems, even after proper introduction and training. Help from relatives or other mantle caregivers may be needed.

Compression therapy should be selected on an individual basis for each patient and each temporary situation. Uniformity of compression device should be considered versus compartmentalization on the limb.

Creative and separate bandaging of each leg "compartment" will eventually result in an acceptable correction of the anatomical contours, rendering maintenance treatment technically feasible.

The effectiveness of compression depends on several technical and personal issues, including the anatomical and functional status of the limb to be treated. There will always be challenging clinical situations where either standard or optimal treatment simply cannot be applied and where clinicians must be creative within the boundaries of their knowledge and expertise. Time and efforts must be invested in finding solutions for applying a sufficient amount of pressure and stiffness while at the same time permitting all activities of daily living.

4.4 Self-Management, Motivation, Adherence, Socio-Cultural and Financial Factors

In venous disease, compression therapy will aim at optimizing venous ambulatory functioning, edema reduction, normalization of secondary skin changes (C4-C6) and relief of subjective symptoms/quality of life. Thus, the patient's lifestyle and concordance will direct the choice of compression device.

The major practical difficulty of compression treatment, and the best predicting factor for ulcer resistance or recurrence is "non-compliance" by the caregiver or the patient, for various reasons. Indeed, the choice of compression regime should be individualised to the temporary needs of each patient. A good function and mobility of the ankle joint must be preserved or restored if possible, since this is a condition sine qua non for calf pump effectiveness.

More than for stockings application of bandages requires learning and training for both the caregiver and the patient.

Nurses must be trained, and physicians must be interested and experienced to ensure correct prescription, follow up, management and coaching of the compression treatment. And people suffering from severe venous insufficiency must be willing to take the responsibility of their own health in a therapeutic partnership [5].

4.5 Availability of Materials, Organization and Provision of Care

The experience and competency of the bandager/care giver, and country-specific factors like availability of materials, reimbursement and national (para-)medical resources will influence cost of treatment and choice of materials.

Often there is a choice between several types of compression devices which are all in principle appropriate for a patient in a given situation. Selection will be based upon the assessment of several parameters as mentioned above, to offer a safe, clinically effective and cost-effective care, well acceptable and to which the patient will be compliant.

In some countries more than in others, there is a wide choice of bandaging materials and therapeutic elastic hosiery, of which timing and application technique must be fitted to the individual patient's temporary needs. Indications and contra-indications exist for both elastic and non-elastic materials and techniques.

Professionals should learn how to use the respective technical advantages of the several systems to the profit of the patient [6].

Short stretch compression is preferred by many in the case of deep venous reflux, phleboedema, lipodermatosclerosis, or for starting up a therapy phase, all in mobile patients. The technique is not always easy to learn, and these short stretch bandages slip off more easily especially when effective in removing edema. Even when they do stay on, the pressure drops within a few hours, but the pressure wave "amplitude" remains in the effective range. This is sometimes cumbersome, requiring more frequent re-application of the bandage. Their advantage lies in the well tolerated low resting pressure (in the supine position) and the high pressure-peaks during activity. It must be underlined that the initially exerted pressure of any bandage system depends more on the application technique (the hand of the person who applies it) than on the technical characteristics of the bandage roll.

Long stretch bandages and elastic stockings are easier to apply and to learn for self-care. Sustained higher pressure values may reach a level of risk in case of excessive force on top of bony prominences or tendons, and there for the stockings or elastic bandages must be removed at night. Special attention is needed in case of arteriopathy, microangiopathy, diabetes, or hypertension.

Another advantage of bandages in general is the fact that they will always fit the leg whatever happens to volume or configuration. Superposition of elastic materials can reach the same degree of stiffness and effectiveness since the successive spires or superposed layers of fabric limit each others' expansion. This effect is amplified when using cohesive or adhesive bandages, which can be left in place for several days, and are good choice for ambulatory patients who are unable to care for compression themselves. The option is then to leave the ulcerated area reachable for daily care or to enclose it in the sustained bandage. Often, availability of care and follow-up will be a decisive factor in making choices. The same holds for organisation of care, reimbursement of provision of care and materials used.

Another important factor to consider is the durability of the materials (wear and tear, deterioration and damage from continued use) in countries with a challenging climate and poor availability of materials or paucity of trained caregivers.

In such circumstances it is worth considering if the whole limb can be treated with one single technique during all phases of wound healing.

Professionals should learn how to use the respective technical advantages of available materials to the profit of the patient [6]. Indications and contra-indications exist for both elastic and non-elastic materials and techniques [7].

Aspects to consider are frequency of application, constant elastic pressure or varying resting and working pressures, and additional therapeutic measures including elevation of the legs, mobilization exercises, assistance devices to don the stockings, protective padding, and footwear.

Assistance devices facilitate the donning of stockings, especially when these are prescribed in superposition, and these should be prescribed, and their usage explained to the patients, for this may substantially enhance compliance and self-care.

Inelastic bandages are classically recommended in the initial phase of treatment. In many cases, these need to be reapplied (preferably by trained staff) since they quickly lose pressure following application. Specialized personnel are not always available and the need to employ them understandably increases cost of treatment for health care service and patients alike.

Self-adjustable compression wrap devices are a welcome well tolerated alternative to bandages since they allow self-application and self-treatment. Research has demonstrated that they may be used in the initial and maintenance stages of compression treatment [8]. Readjusting them maintains high pressure and stiffness over time. The fact that they are reusable reduces the cost of treatment regarding materials [8, 9]. Their effectiveness in healing venous leg ulcers have been demonstrated [8, 10].

Finally, the importance of good footwear must not be underestimated: good quality shoes provide a sustained non-elastic support for the foot and sometimes even the ankle, complementing bandages or stockings worn on the leg. Unfortunately, in challenging climatological and economical situations, shoes are not worn by many of the patients.

4.6 Future Developments, Research Needed

Traditionally, compression extends to the base of the toes. In warm and humid tropical climates shoes are either very limited or not worn at all. Slippers or similar minimal foot protection is preferred instead. Dust, mud, passages through water loops, rocky or stony ground all impact on durability of compression materials. In patients suffering from venous disease this represents an extra challenge since most of the area around the ankles is the zone to be compressed if there is an ulcer or skin changes due to venous disease. Working circumstances may be such that wearing compression bandage or stockings including the foot is a problem, e.g. in muddy ground, rice fields, mines, or when work entails climbing ladders or trees.

New insights stress that the calf muscle pump is the largest venous blood pool to be emptied by compression treatment; more research needs to focus on the necessity to compress the foot if a solution can be found to treat the ankle area. Or to use cheap, separate, easily renewable foot and ankle parts. In a study evaluating an adjustable compression device in venous edema, distal swelling of the ankle and foot was not observed, despite high pressure on the leg. A half stocking was enough to prevent swelling of the most distal parts [8].

Sweating may be another reason for not wearing compression, at least not during the day. With limited modalities for washing and drying fabrics, skin maceration and infection constitute a risk. Washing will shorten durability of any compression device, and manufacturers usually inform the user about this aspect. Compression materials containing elastic fibres may deteriorate more quickly in humid sunny circumstances as well, while inelastic stiff materials are potential hazardous in terms of causing friction and other injury of the skin, as well as slipping down due to loss of pressure or lack of conformability.

Textile research and developments is an interesting field to follow-up concerning future evolutions in compression bandages and stockings. Textile fibers specially adapted to hot humid climates, to intense wear and tear, are mandatory for tropical regions. New fibers, fabric enhancement regarding durability or antiseptic properties are examples of future interests. Smart textiles must be developed that would monitor pressures or other biological parameters, to assess treatment adherence.

Not only the technical characteristics of compression materials must be considered, the anatomical morphological data must be checked to make sure "European" standard sizes will fit the target population.

4.7 Conclusion

Guidelines and recommendations on compression treatment are based on experimental studies and evidence-based insights in the hemodynamic and physiological effects of applying pressure to limbs and other body parts. In clinical practice, some patients do not fit in the routine treatment algorithms.

To be effective and to stimulate compliance, it is interesting to choose the optimal treatment best adapted to the actual needs of the individual patient.

Some rules of the game must be followed to reach our purpose to heal a venous ulcer, normalize the skin changes, and prevent recurrence.

Relying on experience and expertise, caregivers will then need creative solutions to accommodate odd leg shapes or heterogenous tissue consistency. Combining the advantages and effectiveness of different materials and application methods on different parts of a diseased limb is one way to overcome deterioration of skin changes in these patients. Since there are no validated recommendations to guide us in these exceptionally severe cases, it is wise to record and document in the patient's file the materials and techniques used, and the achieved treatment outcomes. The responsibility for potential side-effects indeed lies with the care-giver, therefore improvising "variations on a theme" should remain in the hands of a trained and experienced person.

References

1. Ramelet AA, Perrin M, Kern P, Bounameaux H. Phlebology. 5th ed. Masson: Elsevier; 2008.
2. National Health and Nutrition Examination Survey. www.cdc.gov/nchs/nhanes.htm.
3. Mosti G, De Maeseneer M, Cavezzi A, Parsi K, Morrison N, Nelzen O, Rabe E, Partsch H, Caggiati A, Simka M, Obermayer A, Malouf M, Flour M, Maleti O, Perrin M, Reina L, Kalodiki E, Mannello F, Rerkasem K, Cornu-Thenard A, Chi YW, Soloviy M, Bottini O, Mendyk N, Tessari L, Varghese R, Etcheverry R, Pannier F, Lugli M, Carvallo Lantz AJ, Zamboni P, Zuolo M, Godoy MF, Godoy JM, Link DP, Junger M, Scuderi A. Society for Vascular Surgery and

American Venous Forum Guidelines on the management of venous leg ulcers: the point of view of the International Union of Phlebology. Int Angiol. 2015;34(3):202–18.
4. Eklöf B, Bergan JJ, Carpentier PH, et al. Revision of the CEAP classification for chronic venous disorders. A consensus statement. J Vasc Surg. 2004;40:1248–52.
5. Raju S, Hollis K, Neglen P. Use of compression stockings in chronic venous disease: patient compliance and efficacy. Ann Vasc Surg. 2007;21(6):790–5.
6. Neumann HA, Cornu-Thénard A, Jünger M, Mosti G, Munte K, Partsch H, Rabe E, Ramelet AA, Streit M. Evidence-based (S3) guidelines for diagnostics and treatment of venous leg ulcers. J Eur Acad Dermatol Venereol. 2016. https://doi.org/10.1111/jdv.1_13848.
7. Partsch H, Flour M, Coleridge Smith P, et al. Indications for compression therapy in venous and lymphatic disease. Consensus based on experimental data and scientific evidence. Under the auspices of the IUP. Int Angiol. 2008;27:193–219.
8. Mosti G, Cavezzi A, Partsch H, Urso S, Campana F. Adjustable Velcro® compression devices are more effective than inelastic bandages in reducing venous edema in the initial treatment phase: a randomized controlled trial. Eur J Vasc Endovasc Surg. 2015;50:368–74.
9. Williams A. A review of the evidence for adjustable compression wrap devices. J Wound Care. 2016 May;25(5):242–7. https://doi.org/10.12968/jowc.2016.25.5.242.
10. Blecken SR, Villaviciencio JL, Kao TC. Comparison of elastic versus nonelastic compression in bilateral venous ulcers: a randomized trial. J Vasc Surg. 2005;42:1150–5.

Chapter 5
Surgical Solutions Are an Alternative to Compression Bandaging in Venous Leg Ulcer

Boonying Siribumrungwong, Saritphat Orrapin, Raj Mani, and Kittipan Rerkasem

Abstract Venous leg ulcer is an important health problem worldwide in which compression therapy has been recommended as first line standard treatment. However, some patients fail after compression therapy or have poor compliance with it. In this chapter, we discussed about other alternative treatments especially surgical therapy along with theirs evidence-based recommendations according to pathophysiology of venous leg ulcer.

Keywords Venous ulcer · Endovenous · Compression · Compliance

5.1 Pathophysiology

Skin and subcutaneous tissues are target organs being affected in chronic venous disease (CVD), resulting from repeated injury and inflammation secondary to venous hypertension in the upright position. In the supine position, lower leg venous pressure is approximately 15 mmHg higher than right atrium causing cephalad venous flow toward heart. The pressure is transmitted from residual pressure of capillary bed. However, in upright position, venous pressure rises about 0.8 mmHg

B. Siribumrungwong · S. Orrapin
Faculty of Medicine, Division of Vascular and Endovascular Surgery, Department of Surgery, Thammasat University Hospital, Thammasat University, Pathum Thani, Thailand

R. Mani
Academic Division of Human Health and Development, Faculty of Medicine, University of Southampton, Southampton, UK

Faculty of Medicine, Chiang Mai University, Chiang Mai, Thailand

Shanghai Jiao Tong University School of Medicine, Shanghai, China

K. Rerkasem (✉)
Faculty of Medicine, Division of Vascular and Endovascular Surgery, Department of Surgery, Chiang Mai University, Chiang Mai, Thailand

R. Mani et al. (eds.), *Compression and Chronic Wound Management*,
https://doi.org/10.1007/978-3-030-01195-6_5

for every 1 cm underneath right atrium from hydrostatic pressure of venous column in venous system, resulting in rising of ankle venous pressure to 50–60 and 80–100 mmHg in sitting and standing positions respectively. Pumping mechanisms from synchronized muscle contraction of foot, calf, and thigh during ambulation (also called as secondary heart) help squeezing venous blood toward heart with venous valve preventing reversal of blood flow. These mechanisms cause falling of venous pressure during ambulation (Fig. 5.1) [1]. In normal subjects, the ankle

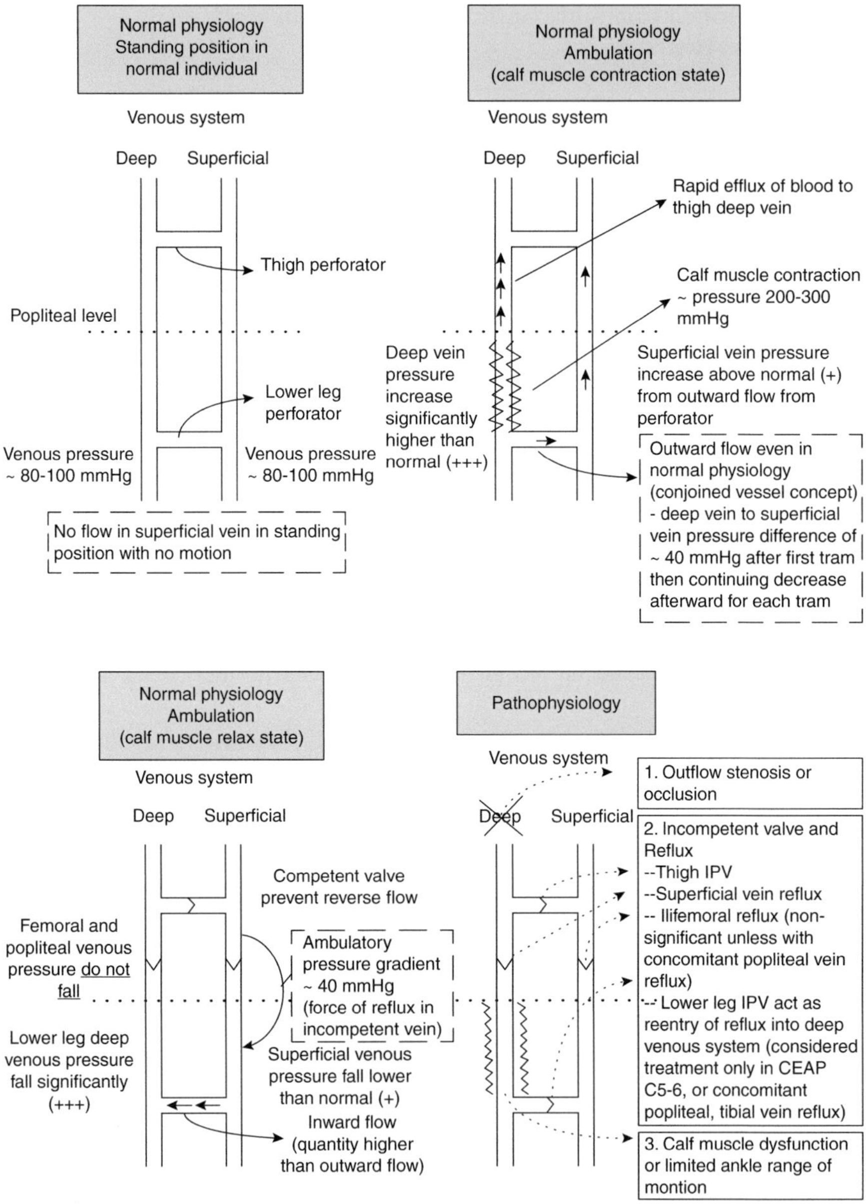

Fig. 5.1 Normal physiology and pathophysiology in chronic venous disease

venous pressure fall to ~25 (SD = 4.9) mmHg during ambulation and slowly rising after cessation of muscle contraction from refilling of blood from capillaries bed [2]. Ambulatory venous hypertension is defined as absence of physiologic pressure fall in the lower leg vein during calf muscle contraction [3].

Factors causing impairment of these mechanisms resulting in ambulatory venous hypertension are venous outflow obstruction, valvular incompetence, calf muscle dysfunction, and limited ankle motion in which valvular incompetence being the most frequent causes [3]. Venous hypertension leads to chronic endothelial injury of capillaries; resulting in leakage of red blood cells, macromolecules, plasma, and fibrinogen into the interstitial space, triggering inflammatory response in the surrounding tissues [4, 5]. As a result, in the lower calf area, changes occur leading to hyperpigmentation and lipodermatosclerosis predisposing skin over the ankles to venous ulceration. Advanced CVD (CEAP C4–6) patients had significant higher ambulatory pressure compared to CEAP C1–3 [2]. Several inflammatory cytokines (e.g. vascular endothelial growth factor, tumor necrosis factor alpha, and interleukin-1) in venous ulcer tissue had been demonstrated to decrease after treatment [6]. With difference pathophysiology causing venous hypertension, duplex scan should be done in every individual patient to identify site of occlusion and reflux patterns that should be considered to be corrected [7]. Ilio-caval occlusive lesion should be suspected in CEAP C3 or higher in whom not response to standard treatment [8].

5.2 Compression Therapy Mechanisms

Compression therapy is a mainstay treatment of venous ulcer and being recommended as initial standard treatment [7, 9]. Compression exerts its effects in two parts; (1) by reducing ambulatory venous pressure in both patients with superficial and deep venous insufficiency [10]. Compression reduces ambulatory venous hypertension by increase ejection fraction of the calf muscle, decrease reflux of superficial vein by narrowing lumen of the vein, and decrease residual venous volume of leg [10, 11] and (2) raising interstitial tissue pressure by directly compression at the ulcer and surrounding tissue, and consequently reduces oedema [12] and might decreased macromolecule leakages. This mechanism acted directly to target organ of CVD, and might explained the microcirculatory beneficial effects of compression therapy that could not be totally explained by improvement of hemodynamic change that occur after only superficial reflux ablation alone [13].

5.3 Limitation of Compression Therapy

5.3.1 Compression Therapy and Compliance

Compliance is the utmost important factor for the effectiveness of compression therapy because its' effect occurs only when putting on as a level I evidence in a consensus document [14]. In non-compliant patients, the healing rate of venous ulcer was lower and time to heal was about 2 months slower than compliant ones [15, 16]. Moreover, rate of recurrence was higher in non-compliant patients [15–17]. However, compliance is low as demonstrated by only 21–37% of patients using it regularly. Pain and discomfort were main factors of non-compliant. Others causes were intangible sense of restriction, lack of advice, and application difficulties and so on. Patients also complaint of the excessive heat in hot and humid climates. Costs of compression therapy should also be considered in developing countries [18, 19]. Unfortunately, several interventions (e.g. socialization, counseling, behavior modification, and nurse-led-self-management program) were proposed to improve compliance, however, no any rigorous evidence to support their efficacies [20].

5.3.2 Compression Therapy and Peripheral Arterial Disease

Peripheral arterial disease (PAD) occurs simultaneously with venous ulcer in approximately 15–25% [21]. Ankle brachial index (ABI) should be measured in every venous ulcer patients to identify patients with PAD [7, 14, 22]. In severe PAD (ABI <0.5 or absolute ankle pressure <60 mmHg), revascularization should be considered. For PAD with ABI of 0.5–0.85, modified compression with ankle pressure of 30 mmHg with regular follow up could be done with minimal risk. However, the healing rate was significantly lower than patients with no PAD. Compression therapy was also has limitation in patients with leg bypass graft [22].

5.3.3 Failure to Heal

Although compression therapy is the mainstay treatment in venous ulcer, significant number of venous ulcer failed to heal with compression therapy alone with the failure rate of 12–40% [23, 24]. Risk factors for failure were reduced ankle range of motion, larger wound area, non-compliance, history of deep venous thrombosis and duration of wound [24–26]. After initiation of compression therapy, assessment of compliance should be done and response to treatment should be objectively documented every 4–6 weeks. In poor compliance or non-response patients, cause of non-compliance or non-improvement should be looked for and managed, sometimes repeated or more investigations should be done. Other adjunctive treatment such as split thickness skin graft should be considered [7, 27]. Although, compression has been the mainstay of treatment, it had high recurrence rate (~50%) when used as a sole therapy in long-term follow up. Eradication of cause of ambulatory venous hypertension should be done.

5.4 Others Treatment Modalities

Other modalities to treat venous ulcer can be classified according to their pathophysiology of venous ulcer. Grading of recommendation and evidences supported of their efficacies are summarized in Table 5.1.

Table 5.1 Treatment modalities other than compression therapy to manage venous leg ulcer according to pathophysiology with guideline evidences

Pathophysiology	Treatment	Evidences and grade of recommendation
Reduce ambulatory venous hypertension		
Outflow occlusion		
Iliac vein stenosis or occlusion	– Endovascular angioplasty and stenting – Open bypasses procedure (after failed endovascular treatment and recalcitrant ulcer) – Deep venous obstruction should be treated first, before considering treatment of deep venous reflux	1C[a]; Class IIa, B[b] 2C[a] Class I, C[b]
Infrainguinal stenosis or occlusion	– Endophlebectomy, or autogenous venous bypass (only in recalcitrant ulcer) to aid healing and prevent recurrence	2C[a]
Valvular incompetence and reflux		
Deep venous reflux	– Valve repair (external banding, external, and internal valvuloplasty), valve transposition or transplantation – In the absence of deep venous obstruction, and after abolition of superficial venous reflux, open repair of deep venous reflux in severe CVD should be considered	2C[a] Class IIb, C[b]
Superficial venous reflux with active venous ulcer	– Ablation to aid ulcer healing – Ablation to prevent recurrence	2C[a] 1B[a]
Superficial venous reflux with healed venous ulcer	– Ablation to prevent recurrence	1C[a]
GSV reflux	– Endothermal ablation is preferred over surgery and foam sclerotherapy	Class I, A[b]
SSV reflux	– Endothermal ablation should be considered	Class IIa, B[b]
Pathologic perforator in CEAP C5–6	– Ablation to aid ulcer healing and prevent recurrence in pathologic perforator with/without superficial reflux – Percutaneous technique is preferred over open surgery	2C[a] 1C[a]
Calf muscle function and limited ankle range of motion	– Supervised exercise to reduce pain and edema	2B[a]

(continued)

Table 5.1 (continued)

Pathophysiology	Treatment	Evidences and grade of recommendation
Local inflammatory effects		
Micronized purified flavonoid fraction or pentoxifylline	– Should be combined treatment with compression therapy to fasten and aid in ulcer healing	1B[a]
Sulodexide and micronized purified flavonoid fraction	– Should be considered as adjuvant therapy in venous ulcer	Class IIa, A[b]
Other modalities		
Split-thickness skin grafting	– In selected patients with large ulcer that failed conservative treatment for 4–6 weeks	2B[a]
Leg elevation	– May be considered when compression is not tolerated and in conjunction with compression during resting	Class IIb, C[b]

[a]Clinical practice guidelines of the Society for Vascular Surgery and the American Venous Forum 2014 [7]. Grade of recommendation: 1 = strong, 2 = weak recommendation. Level of evidence: A = high; B = moderate, C = low quality

[b]Clinical practice guidelines of the European Society for Vascular Surgery 2015 [9]. Class of recommendation: I = treatment beneficial, recommended, II = conflicting evidences and/or divergence opinion, IIa = favor of usefulness and efficacy, IIb = usefulness/efficacy is less well established, III = treatment not useful, not recommended. Level of evidence: A = from meta-analysis or multiple randomized controlled trials. B = single randomized controlled trial, or large nonrandomized studies. C = Consensus, retrospective studies, or registries

5.4.1 Outflow Occlusion

Outflow occlusion (or stenosis) of venous flow from lower leg can be classified according to level of diseases; (1) ilio-caval level which involve iliac vein and inferior vena cava and (2) infra-inguinal level which involve femoral, popliteal and tibial veins.

5.4.1.1 Ilio-Caval Vein Stenosis or Occlusion

Ilio-caval vein lesions can be occurred after deep vein thrombosis (post-thrombotic syndrome) or from external compression (non-thrombotic iliac vein lesions (NIVLs)). Iliac vein lesion is the significant cause of CVD with the prevalence of 20% in two recent studies [28, 29]. After iliofemoral vein thrombosis, 70% of patients recanalised incompletely resulting in residual occlusion with marked ambulatory venous hypertension [30]. NIVLs are fibrotic or membranous stenosis that believed to be caused from repeated injury from arterial pulsation nearby. Pathology of NIVLs included focal strictures, trabecular strands, and membranes that may present with or without deep vein thrombosis [8]. When combining with deep vein reflux, outflow occlusion is considered as predominant hemodynamic significant lesion and should be treated first. Intravascular ultrasound (IVUS) was the gold standard to diagnose significant iliac vein lesion since femoral venography and computed tomographic venography were insensitive. In addition, IVUS should be

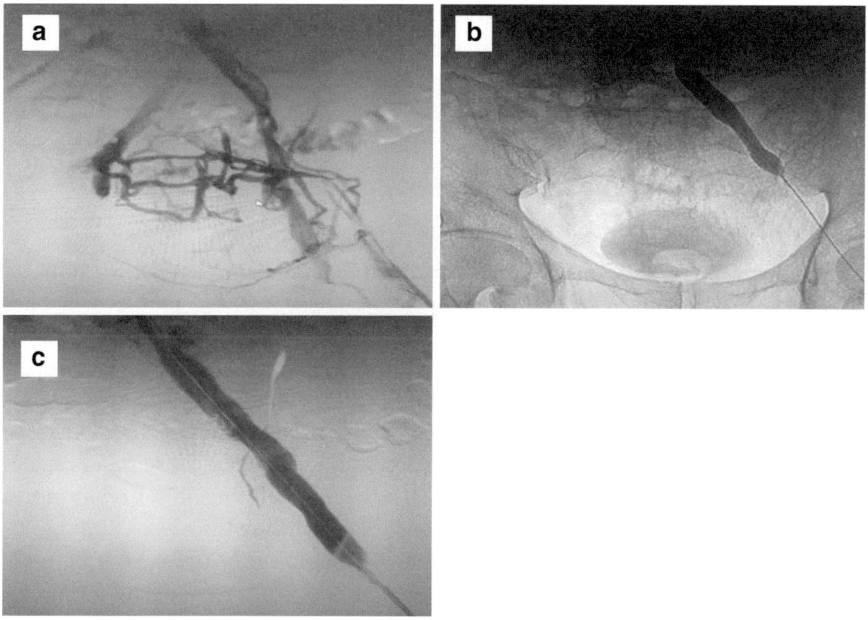

Fig. 5.2 Iliac vein occlusion in venous ulcer patient. (**a**) Venogram found stenosis and marked collaterals seen; (**b**) balloon venoplasty; (**c**) venogram after venoplasty and stent placement found abscence of collaterals. Technical consideration [7]: (i) Large bore stent is mandatory in all cases to prevent recoil from fibrosis (Inferior vena cava—20 mm, common iliac vein 16 mm. external iliac vein 14 mm, and common femoral vein 12 mm). (ii) Avoid skip area to prevent residual lesion and interstent stenosis. (iii) Proximal extension of stent usually be placed 2–3 cm above iliac vein bifurcation into inferior vena cava to prevent squeezing of the stent distally. (iv) Intravascular ultrasound is useful to located proper position of stent and lesion coverage

performed during intervention to help delineate extension and complete coverage of the lesion after stenting [31].

Endovascular angioplasty with mandatory stenting is the standard treatment in ilio-caval vein lesions. The success rate was 97.6% with cumulative patency of 90–100% and 74–83% for non-thrombotic and post-thrombotic disease at 3–5 year respectively, see Fig. 5.2 [8, 9]. Treatment resulted in relief of pain and improvement of quality of life in most patients and persistent healing of venous ulcer in 56–100% in recalcitrant ulcer despite in patients with combined deep venous reflux [9, 32]. Open surgical bypasses (e.g. femoro-iliac-caval bypass, femoro-femoral bypass with using vein (Palma procedures) might be considered only in recalcitrant venous ulcer with failed endovascular procedure [9].

5.4.1.2 Infrainguinal Occlusive Lesions

Infrainguinal reconstruction included endophlebectomy (surgical disobliteration of postthrombotic vein) and autogenous venous bypass. Success depends on adequate venous inflow, outflow, and use of autogenous vein. The success rate varies between

40% and 60% at 2–4 years [7, 9]. However, most reported studies were small and retrospective with marked variation in techniques and concomitant procedures that are difficult to be validated and concluded [33, 34].

5.4.2 *Valvular Incompetent and Reflux*

Venous reflux is a retrograde venous flow in an incompetent vein during ambulation in upright position. During calf muscle contraction, the pressure in both superficial and deep veins at ankle fall, but not at popliteal and femoral veins. This pressure difference between calf and thigh veins is called ambulatory pressure gradient which is about 30–40 mmHg [35]. Incompetent valves of vein connecting these two poles of pressure gradient cause reflux of venous blood back to the lower leg vein during and at the end of ambulation. Reflux cause rapid returning of ankle venous pressure to resting state (rapid refilling time) resulting in high daily mean ambulatory venous pressure. The refilling time was 31 and 2.8 s in normal subjects and patients with great saphenous vein reflux, respectively [36]. Incompetent valve can be primarily caused from venous dilatation or inflammatory damage of the valve leaflet induced by shear stress; or secondary to post-thrombosis. Treatment of reflux results in decreasing mean daily ambulatory venous hypertension and logically leading to ulcer healing and decrease recurrence [37].

5.4.2.1 Deep Venous Reflux

Site of reflux in deep venous system have been associated with venous hemodynamic significance. Without superficial reflux, popliteal-valve competent prevent reflux of deep venous system down to calf from ambulatory pressure gradient therefore ilio-femoral vein reflux added little to hemodynamic abnormality without presenting of popliteal reflux [1, 3, 38]. These can be demonstrated by restoration of normal venous hemodynamic after superficial reflux ablation in case with concomitant femoral and superficial reflux [39]. Treatment comprises of primary valve repair (external banding, external or internal valvuloplasty), valve transposition, and transplantation in CEAP C5–6 non-response to conservative therapy with competent outflow. Good short-term results are reported with competent rate of 50–60% at 60 months follow up and ulcer healing rate of 54–60% at 5 years [7, 9]. Their efficacy have been shown in both primary reflux and postthrombotic syndrome. Internal valvuloplasty is the treatment of choice in primary reflux whereas valve transposition, transplantation, and replacement valves have been considered in post-thrombotic syndrome [40–42]. However, these solutions are technically demanding with no guarantee of success.

5.4.2.2 Superficial Venous Reflux

Two main superficial venous system are great saphenous vein (GSV) and short saphenous vein (SSV) in which GSV is the most common site of reflux. Superficial venous reflux ablation had been demonstrated to significantly reduce ambulatory venous pressure [1]. However, it is generally recommended to ablate the refluxed veins after healing of venous ulcer based on results from a RCT (ESCHAR trial) [43] and a systematic review and meta-analysis in 2014 [37]. These two studies demonstrated no benefit of surgical interventions to ulcer healing compared to compression therapy alone, but surgical intervention could reduce long term recurrence after 4 years follow up in ESCHAR trial (51% vs 27%: $p < 0.01$) [43]. Surgeons are also concerned about wound infection when performing open surgery with frank (or open) ulcer.

At present, in the era of minimally invasive surgery, endovenous procedure can be done without incision. A cohort study of endovenous laser ablation (EVLA) in superficial venous reflux with healed or active venous ulcer concluded that EVLA can be safely offered to patients active and healed venous ulcer even the elderly with significant morbidities with low recurrence rate at 3 year [44]. Many new evidence supports benefits of endovenous procedure to ulcer healing and recurrence rather than the use of just compression. Recently, a multicenter RCT including 450 patients with venous leg ulcer demonstrated shorter median time to heal (about 26 days), and longer ulcer-free time at 1 year in the early-intervention group [45]. Another One RCT demonstrated 81.5% ulcer healing rate after EVLA vs. 24% after compression alone at 12 months ($p < 0.001$) with no recurrence after EVLA but 44% in the other group [46]. Other cohort study also found significant higher rate of ulcer healing in endovenous group compared to compression alone (62% vs 36% at 1 year) [47].

Based on these evidence, we concluded that in a patient with a venous leg ulcer and incompetent superficial vein, the ablation of superficial vein without compression therapy can improve ulcer healing and should be done early after diagnosis. This is perhaps being suitable in warm climate in tropical countries, which patients had low compliance for compression therapy. Intervention should be offered concomitantly with compression therapy to aid ulcer healing, prevent recurrence, and reduce overall cost of treatment [48]. Many techniques of endovenous procedure are available with similar aiming at ablation of refluxed vein are summarized here according to site of reflux.

Great Saphenous Vein Reflux

Standard treatment of GSV reflux is endovenous procedures with demonstrated similar efficacies to open surgery except ultrasound-guided foam sclerotherapy which is worst. Causes of recurrence between endovenous procedures and open surgery are different which are incomplete stripping, and neovascularization after surgery whereas reflux in tributaries and recanalization are more common after endovenous procedures [49]. In endovenous procedure, to prevent injury to deep venous system, tip of catheter is usually placed at a few centimeters distal to sapheno-femoral junction leaving tributaries branches to be patent causing more reflux in tributaries afterward while saphenofemoral ligation was ligated flush to common femoral vein in open surgery. Dissection of groin wound had been claimed to associate with neovascularization in open surgery but no dissection necessary in endovenous procedures. Although causes of recurrences are different, it counterbalances to each other, thus result in similar rate of clinical recurrence [50]. Advantages of endovenous procedures over surgery (venous stripping) are less post-procedural pain, fasten recovery, and rapid return to normal activities and work [50, 51].

Endovenous therapy can be classified into endovenous thermal and non-thermal ablation in which mechanisms involve and not involve heat respectively. Endovenous thermal ablation includes endovenous laser ablation (EVLA), radiofrequency ablation (RFA), and steam ablation. Tumescent anesthesia (TA) usually be applied in thermal ablation to prevent adjacent tissue injury from heat. Non-thermal ablation includes ultrasound-guided foam sclerotherapy, mechanicochemical endovenous ablation (MOCA), and cyanoacrylate injection and usually without TA (non-tumescent non-thermal, NTNT).

Radiofrequency Ablation (RFA)

Radiofrequency ablation (RFA; Covidien ClosureFAST™, San Jose, CA, USA) (Fig. 5.3) use a catheter with 7- and 3-cm heating elements that is generated by radiofrequency energy. Ablation will be done segmentally by consistent heat generation to 120 °C for 20 s for each segment. TA is applied with objectives to decrease thermal injury to adjacent tissue, compress and emptying the vein for proper contact of catheter to endothelium, and push skin away from catheter in case of shallow GSV (<1 cm from skin). External compression using ultrasound probe during heat generation is also recommended to achieve vein occlusion [52].

Endovenous Laser Ablation (EVLA)

EVLA using laser energy to generate heat. Several technical factors have been associated with efficacies including wavelength, pulsed vs continuous wave, power, and pull back speed. Laser energy with shorter wavelengths (e.g. 810, 940, and 980 nm) are absorbed by hemoglobin and converted to heat, producing steam of bubbles that distribute along and injure the endothelial wall. Catheter tip temperature of 800 °C had been reported with occasionally caused vein wall perforation and ecchymosis. Longer wavelength laser (e.g. 1470, 1560 nm) is less absorbed by hemoglobin but absorbed by water in the vein wall that may increase efficacy with less complication [53, 54].

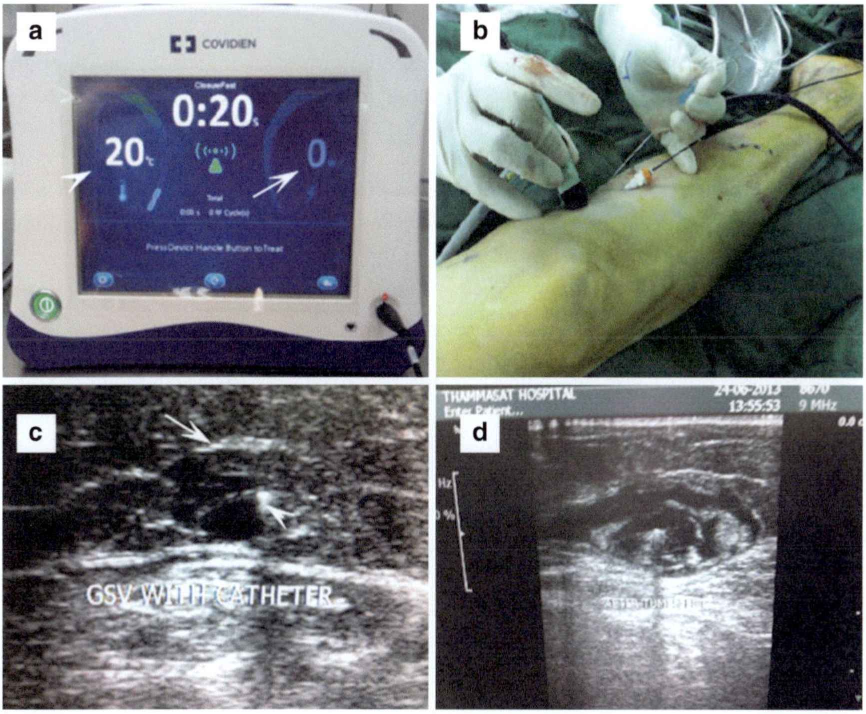

Fig. 5.3 Radiofrequency ablation (ClosureFast™ catheter) of great saphenous vein reflux. (**a**) RF generator; arrowhead demonstrates temperature at tip of the catheter, arrow demonstrate power usage as Watt (W). Usually power will begin at ~40 W then gradually drop to below 20 W within 10 s. If the temperature is not reached to 120 °C within 5 s or the power stay about 20 W, there may be some flow within the vein. (**b**) Tumescent anesthesia (TA). (**c**) RFA catheter in the GSV; arrowhead demonstrate catheter, arrow demonstrate saphenous fascia. (**d**) Circumferential fluid layer of TA around the vein. GSV is collapsed allowing direct contact of vein endothelium to the heating elements. Approximately volume of 10 cc/cm of vein is recommended. Hint. Catheter tip position should be confirmed before TA. TA should be done at the saphenofemoral junction to limit flow from tributaries and to completely compress the GSV beyond catheter tip to prevent injury from heating fluid that go 1–1.5 cm further from the tip of the catheter

Endovenous Steam Ablation (EVSA)

This procedure also use heat from steam to ablate GSV. Venous cannulation and TA are applied as other endovenous procedures. The catheter has two radial opposite holes at tip to emit steam. The steam generator will heat sterile pressurized water to 150 °C by an electrical current. At the tip of catheter, the pulse steam will dispel the condensate water out of the catheter. Three pulses are applied at the most proximal GSV (2–3 cm from saphenofemoral junction) then 2–4 pulses for every 1-cm vein segment [55].

Ultrasound-Guided Foam Sclerotherapy (UGFS)

Sclerosant is chemical agent to damage endothelium after injection, endothelium damage cause platelet activation and thrombus formation. Foam can be obtained by mixing liquid sclerosant with air. The most frequently used method to produce foam is Tessari's technique, by rapid mixing 1 cc of liquid sclerosant with 4 cc of air 10–20 times between two connected syringes via a three-way stopcock. Foam sclerosant has higher efficacy than liquid sclerosant and is injected to GSV by direct puncture or via catheter under ultrasound guidance [55].

Mechanico-Chemical Ablation (MOCA)

MOCA using Clarivein® (Vascular Insights LLC, Quincy, MA) is a heatless technique (NTNT) to occlude target vein by simultaneously do both mechanical injury to the vein and sclerotherapy. Clarivein® catheter tip is angled with a metal ball attached to a wire. A wire is connected to battery-motorized handle. A motor will spin the tip of the wire to cause injury to the endothelium and venous spasm while physician simultaneously withdraw the catheter and injected liquid sclerosant [56]. Mechanical injury damage to the media of the vein wall allowing deeper penetration of the sclerosant explaining why its efficacy is better than UGFS [57].

Cyanoacrylate Injection (Fig. 5.4)

Cyanoacrylate injection (VenaSeal; Sapheon, Inc., Morrisville, NC) is a NTNT procedure to occlude GSV by injecting cyanoacrylate (glue) specifically desired for venous intervention via endovenous catheter. After being contacted with blood, cyanoacrylate polymerize into solid form, triggering inflammatory response and fibrosis resulting in vein occlusion [58]. Glue can migrate 2 cm proximally from a compression point therefore it is recommended to place the tip of the catheter about 5 cm from the saphenofemoral junction. Post-procedure compression stocking also not necessary after glue injection. Thrombophlebitis is the most complication after glue injection [59].

All endovenous procedures seem to have similar high occlusion rate except for UGFS which is clearly worse than open surgery [50]. A systematic review and meta-analysis of long-term outcomes (5 year follow up) demonstrated non-different rate of recurrence between RFA, EVLA and surgery [60]. RFA and UGFS had been demonstrated to caused significant less post-procedural pain than EVLA with short wavelength. This can be explained by more heat generated after EVLA with some perforation [50, 61]. However, new generation of EVLA with longer wavelength has been introduced and claimed to have less post-procedural pain than previous ones [62]. Although UGFS had worst efficacy with higher rate of re-intervention, it is cheap and easily repeatable.

A systematic review and meta-analysis of MOCA and glue injection demonstrated pooled anatomical success after MOCA and glue to be 94.7% and 94.8% at 6 month and 94.1% and 89.0% at 1 year, respectively [63]. Early result of a RCT

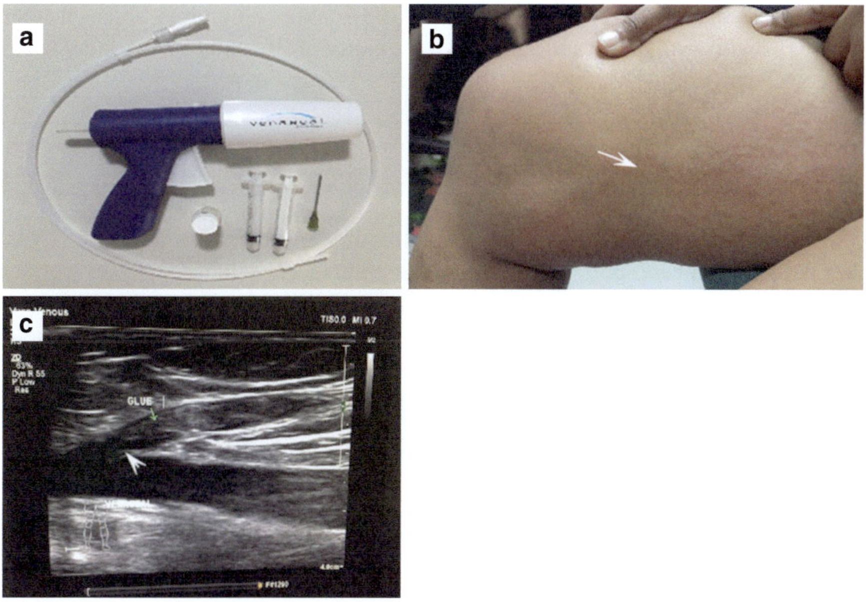

Fig. 5.4 Cyanoacrylate injection in great saphenous vein (GSV) reflux. (**a**) VenaSeal™ Closure System (**b**) Thrombophlebitis of thigh GSV few days after cyanoacrylate injection. It resolved after few-day treatment with oral NSAIDs. (**c**) Glue in GSV nearly enter into common femoral vein (arrow head) from proximal migration. Technical consideration: (i) Avoid kinking of the delivery catheter after filling with glue. (ii) Catheter tip should be placed 5 cm distal to the saphenofemoral junction. (iii) Ultrasound probe compression in transverse plane to completely occlude the GSV just proximal to the delivery catheter during first injection is important to prevent proximal glue migration. (iv) Tip of the delivery catheter should be located after each injection for guide accurate compression point for next injection. (v) The catheter should be remove rapidly after completion of the procedure to prevent adhesion to the skin

comparing MOCA and RFA found similar occlusion rate (92%) at 4 week with less procedural and post-procedural pain with MOCA [64]. A RCT comparing glue vs. RFA (VeClose trial) demonstrated non-inferiority of glue compared to RFA with occlusion rate of 99% for glue and 96% for RFA at 3 months with less post-procedural ecchymosis [65]. However, application could be done only in patients with GSV $\leq$ 12 mm that was the inclusion criteria of the study whereas RFA had been proven to be effective even in vein larger than 12 mm with occlusion rate of 100% at 6 months in group with mean GSV diameter of 17 (SD 4) mm [66]. Although NTNT appear to be safe and effective with less procedural associated pain, more data from long-term follow up study should affirm this findings before making a conclusion.

Cost consideration is also important in countries where endovenous procedures are not reimbursed. Cost-utility study in Thailand in which cost of catheter of endovenous procedures (RFA, EVLA, MOCA, and cyanoacrylate injection) are not reimbursed, revealed that UGFS is the most cost-effective procedure compared with RFA and open surgery even though it had higher re-intervention rate.

The reasons behind the conclusion were UGFS is about a hundred times cheaper than RFA with similar advantages of better quality of life and less workday leave over open surgery [67].

Small Saphenous Vein (SSV) Reflux

SSV reflux account for about 10–15% of reflux site. Treatment is ligation of SSV at 3–5 cm from sapheno-popliteal junction using ultrasound-guided for marking site for incision [51]. Stripping of the SSV may be failed due to complex anatomy. Recently, endovascular therapy has also been performed in SSV reflux with a tendency towards better results compared with surgery [68, 69]. Ablation of SSV by endothermal procedures should not extend below midcalf due to high incidence of paresthesia [9].

5.4.2.3 Perforator Reflux

Calf perforator veins act as a conjoined vessel between tibial veins and superficial veins. Bidirectional flow occurs even in normal subjects causing identical pressure between lower leg deep and superficial veins at rest, ambulation, and recovery periods [3]. Incompetent perforator veins (IPVs) is defined as perforator vein with an outward flow duration of ≥0.5 s, with a diameter ≥3.5 cm and located beneath healed or open venous ulcer [51]. As previously described, reflux occurs in incompetent vein from ambulatory pressure gradient between thigh and calf veins during ambulation. Therefore, calf IPVs usually acts as reentry point of superficial reflux because it locates in the lower pole of the pressure gradient. In case without concomitant deep venous reflux, the net flow of the bidirectional flow in calf IPVs is inward into deep venous system, therefore treatment is not indicated [1, 3]. However, ablation is indicated in IPVs with severe CVI, concomitant popliteal/tibial venous reflux, or thigh IPVs that located at the higher-pressure pole and act as source of reflux. Ablation can improve venous hemodynamic in these IPVs which are called pathologic perforators [7, 51].

Ablation can be done either by surgery (i.e., subfascial endoscopic perforator surgery (SEPS), and modified Linton's procedure) or percutaneously. Pathologic perforator is ligated via endoscope in SEPS whereas it is ligated just above fascia level in modified Linton's procedure using ultrasound-guided incision. However, percutaneous ablation either by ultrasound-guided sclerotherapy or endothermal ablation is recommended to prevent incision on the damaged skin in advanced CVD [70]. Percutaneous access is challenged especially in tortuous one. Tip of endothermal catheter should be placed at least 0.5 cm from the deep parent vein to prevent injury. TA should be applied. Initial success rate after percutaneous ablation varies between 50% and 70%, repeated procedure is common. Successful ablation was associated with ulcer healing in recalcitrant ones [71–73] (Fig. 5.5).

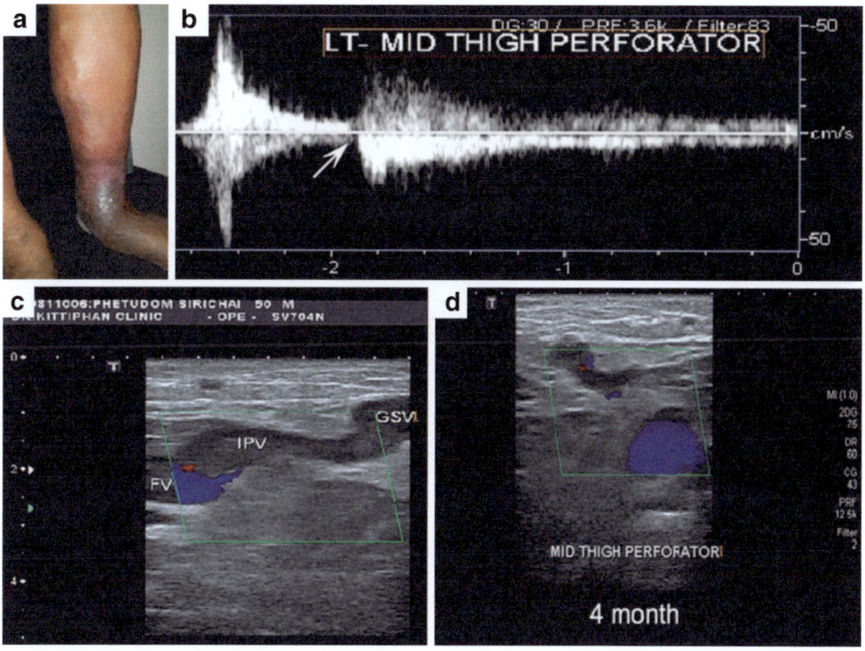

Fig. 5.5 Percutaneous ablation of perforators (PAPs). (**a**) A 57 year old CVO patient with lipodermatosclerosis, and hyperpigmentation. (**b**, **c**) Thigh incompetence perforator vein with diameter of 8 mm demonstrated reverse flow after manual compression and release as was considered as pathologic perforator. Arrow demonstrate point of release after compression. (**d**) Thrombosis of pathologic perforator after percutaneous radiofrequency ablation 4 months

5.4.3 Medication

Systemic drug therapy is prescribed as an adjunct with compression therapy with aim to decrease swelling, pain, and aid ulcer healing. It can be divided into two groups according to their mechanisms of action whether directly related to venous wall or not. Venotonic drugs act directly to venous wall whereas non-venotonic drugs act via other mechanisms. Drugs that had evidenced-based of proven benefit in venous ulcer healing are discussed here which are micronized purified flavonoid fraction (MPFF), sulodexide and pentoxifylline [7, 9].

5.4.3.1 Venotonic Drugs

MPFF exerts their mechanisms via both micro- and macro-circulatory effects. MPFF consists of 90% micronized diosmin and 10% flavonoids. It prevents inflammatory process by inhibition of leukocyte-endothelium interaction resulting in inability of white blood cell to infiltrate venous parenchyma and decreases capillaries permeability. It also increases venous tone via noradrenergic activity extension in smooth muscle cells [74, 75]. MPFF dose is 500 mg twice a day at midday and at mealtimes in evening. Data from meta-analysis demonstrated increase rate of venous ulcer healing with 32% risk reduction (95%CI: 3–70%) with rapid healing time (61.3% vs. 47.7% healing rate at 6 months for MPFF and control groups respectively) [76]. MPFF is also highly effective in improving leg symptoms, edema, and quality of life [77].

Soludexide is a highly-purified glycosaminoglycan with anti-inflammatory, antithrombotic, and profibrinolytic activities. Current systematic review and meta-analysis suggested benefit of increasing rate of ulcer healing (4 RCTs with 463 subjects) with the healing rate of 49.4% vs. 29.8% (Relative risk 1.66; 95%CI: 1.3, 2.1) for soludexide and control respectively. However, the qualities of the evidences were low due to risk of bias, unclear of optimal dosage and frequency, route of administration and its adverse effects [78].

5.4.3.2 Non-venotonic Drugs

Pentoxifylline is a competitive nonselective adenylate cyclase inhibitor results in inhibition of platelet aggregation and thrombus formation and has anti-inflammatory effect via depression of granulocyte phagocytic activity, and neutrophil-endothelium adhesion [79]. Previous evidences from two systematic reviews and meta-analyses demonstrated significant complete healing or significant improvement rate of pentoxifylline (400 mg tablet taken three times a day) compared to placebo with relative risk of 1.7 (95%CI: 1.3, 2.4) [80] and 1.4 (95%CI: 1.3, 1.6) [81].

Low dose aspirin have been administered as adjunctive treatment to compression therapy for venous leg ulcer from possible benefit of its' antiplatelet and antiinflammatory properties. However, its' efficacy was based on low quality evidences [82]. Recently largest RCT including 251 venous ulcers also failed to demonstrate benefit of aspirin [83]. Aspirin, therefore, should not be prescribed to treat venous ulcer from its' unobvious clinical benefit with potential harm.

5.4.4 Calf Muscle Dysfunction and Limited Ankle Mobility

Important factors associated with failure of compression treatment are impairment of calf muscle pump, limited ankle range of motion and poor physical activities (e.g. short walking distance <200 m during the day) [24]. Improvement of calf muscle pump results in increase calf ejection fraction and decrease residual venous volume. A systematic review of 16 studies concluded that increased physical activities, improved mobility and foot exercises as adjunctive treatment of compression therapy could reduce ulcer recurrences [84]. However, recent systematic review of only RCTs found contrast results with no benefit of exercise to calf muscle pump function, ankle range of motion, quality of life and venous ulcer healing rate with possible increase risk of adverse events [85]. Interventions included both supervised structured exercised and home-based exercise programs employing 2–3 times a week for 3–6 months emphasizing on strengthening of calf muscle (e.g. progressive resistance exercise program using heel raise) and stretching of ankle joint (e.g. ankle exercise program using elastic resistance bands and stretching) with 60–90% adherence. Exercise should be done with caution to avoid ankle injury which may limit ambulation [86–89].

5.4.5 *Other Adjunctive Treatments*

5.4.5.1 Patient Counseling and Education

Patient counseling is pivotal to the success of treatment and make good doctor-patient relationship. Patients should understand aims of treatment that are ulcer healing, prevent recurrence afterward, and improve quality of life. Mainstay of treatment is compression therapy and compliance is the utmost important part to achieve the treatment aims and it is patient's responsibility not the doctors'. They should understand that the disease will be better but not cure and it will be last for their lifetime.

5.4.5.2 Wound Care and Split-Thickness Skin Graft (STSG)

Necrotic tissue should be debrided either surgically or by other means such as autolytic debridement, enzymatic debridement, or biological debridement. Surgical debridement should be done with cautious because too deep debridement would remove all adnexal components that are the source of new epithelization. Occlusive dressing should be applied with moist environment to promote autolytic debridement, angiogenesis, and granulation tissue development. Moist assessment and management should be done in every individual wound. In dry wound, hydrogel and hydrocolloid dressing should be applied whereas highly absorbing dressing such as alginates, hydrofibers, or foam are more appropriated in highly exudative wound. Wound edge protection is important in highly exudative wound to prevent edge maceration. Dressing change should be as frequent as required bearing in mind that the ulcer is in proliferative stage and epithelized phase [27, 90].

STSG done using patient's own skin (autograft) or bioengineered skin substitute (allograft) should be considered in venous ulcer that fail to heal with compression therapy especially those with larger wound area (>20 cm^2), deep wound without new islets after treatment, limited ankle range of motion, or non-response to treatment after 4–6 weeks. A systematic review demonstrated healing rate of 73% after STSG [91]. Dermal components of the graft had been shown to improve healing outcomes

[92]. Negative pressure wound therapy had been demonstrated to improve granulation tissue and fasten wound bed preparation for STSG [27].

5.4.5.3 Leg Elevation

An elevation of the affected leg by 10–30 cm above heart level in supine position during the day, before leg compression, at night, or even hospitalization with bed rest could reduce edema, which in turn would increase wound blood flow from decrease pressure at venous end of capillaries and reduction of tissue pressure that might promote venous healing [93, 94]. It should be considered in patients whom cannot tolerate compression from acute painful inflammation, infection, and superficial venous thrombosis. Caution must be exercised to avoid exacerbating effects of reducing after load in elderly patients who may be at risk of right heart failure. Formerly, bed elevation was advised using 9 in. (23 cm) wooden block: compliance with this was variable and this technique would appear to be out of favour. However, leg elevation should be used to reduce edema before bandaging [9].

5.4.5.4 Obesity and Venous Disease

Obese patients seem to have more severe CVI than non-obese with the most common site of reflux was at saphenofemoral junction as in non-obese [95, 96]. Hemodynamic study found greater reflux in obese as seen by decrease venous filling time, and high foot venous pressure than non-obese that might be explained by increase intra-abdominal pressure in obese [97]. At present, no evidence supported that losing weight benefit patients with CVI, however, losing weight by increasing physical activity might help improving calf muscle function and decrease mean daily ambulatory venous pressure with no harm though further study is warranted.

5.5 Conclusion

There are three goals to considered when treating venous ulcer: ulcer healing, prevent recurrences, and improve quality of life. Management requires thorough knowledge and understanding of its' pathophysiology. Compression therapy is mainstay treatment. Accurate investigations to determine causes of venous hypertension is pivotal in decided which interventions will benefit the patients and should be done as soon as possible. To achieve the goals, multidisciplinary approach is required with both non-operative and operative skills. Cooperative and compliance of the patients are other keys to success that may become better by good doctor-patient relationship and understanding of the treatment along with its aims. Diagram of management of venous ulcer is suggested (Fig. 5.6).

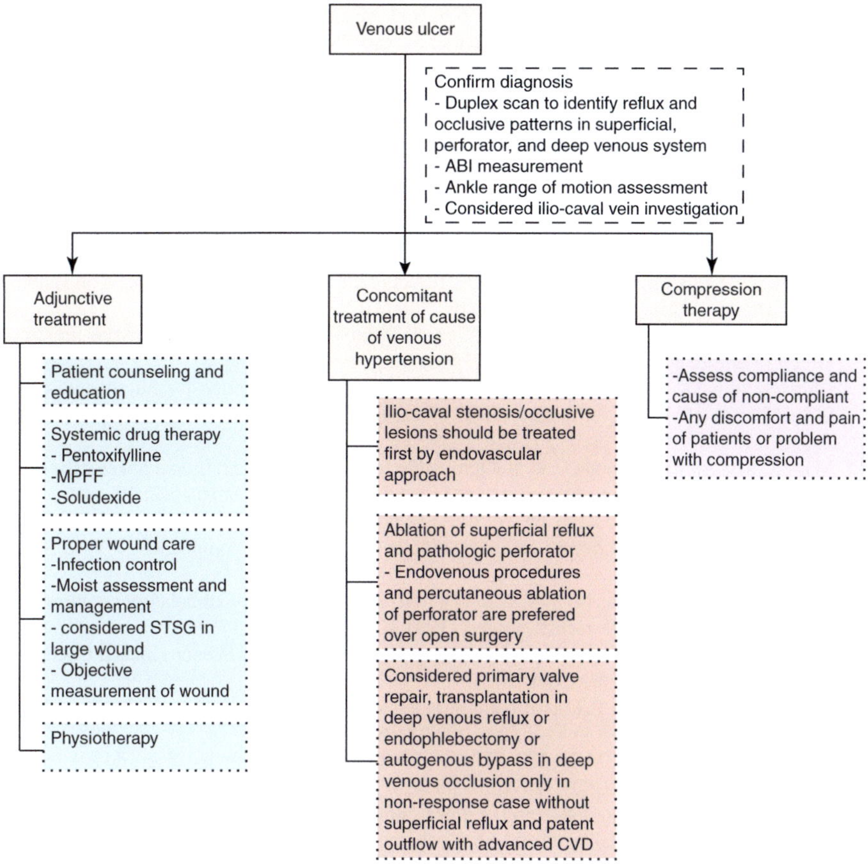

Fig. 5.6 Venous ulcer management conclusion diagram

References

1. Lee BB, Nicolaides AN, Myers K, et al. Venous hemodynamic changes in lower limb venous disease: the UIP consensus according to scientific evidence. Int Angiol. 2016;35(3):236–352.
2. Fukuoka M, Sugimoto T, Okita Y. Prospective evaluation of chronic venous insufficiency based on foot venous pressure measurements and air plethysmography findings. J Vasc Surg. 2003;38(4):804–11.
3. Recek C. Conception of the venous hemodynamics in the lower extremity. Angiology. 2006;57(5):556–63.
4. Virgini-Magalhaes CE, Porto CL, Fernandes FF, et al. Use of microcirculatory parameters to evaluate chronic venous insufficiency. J Vasc Surg. 2006;43(5):1037–44.
5. Bergan JJ, Schmid-Schonbein GW, Smith PD, et al. Chronic venous disease. N Engl J Med. 2006;355(5):488–98.
6. Murphy MA, Joyce WP, Condron C, et al. A reduction in serum cytokine levels parallels healing of venous ulcers in patients undergoing compression therapy. Eur J Vasc Endovasc Surg. 2002;23(4):349–52.

7. O'Donnell TF Jr, Passman MA, Marston WA, et al. Management of venous leg ulcers: clinical practice guidelines of the Society for Vascular Surgery (R) and the American Venous Forum. J Vasc Surg. 2014;60(2 Suppl):3s–59s.
8. Raju S. Treatment of iliac-caval outflow obstruction. Semin Vasc Surg. 2015;28(1):47–53.
9. Wittens C, Davies AH, Baekgaard N, et al. Editor's choice—management of chronic venous disease: clinical practice guidelines of the European Society for Vascular Surgery (ESVS). Eur J Vasc Endovasc Surg. 2015;49(6):678–737.
10. Christopoulos DG, Nicolaides AN, Szendro G, et al. Air-plethysmography and the effect of elastic compression on venous hemodynamics of the leg. J Vasc Surg. 1987;5(1): 148–59.
11. Ibegbuna V, Delis KT, Nicolaides AN, et al. Effect of elastic compression stockings on venous hemodynamics during walking. J Vasc Surg. 2003;37(2):420–5.
12. Nehler MR, Moneta GL, Woodard DM, et al. Perimalleolar subcutaneous tissue pressure effects of elastic compression stockings. J Vasc Surg. 1993;18(5):783–8.
13. Christopoulos DC, Nicolaides AN, Belcaro G, et al. Venous hypertensive microangiopathy in relation to clinical severity and effect of elastic compression. J Dermatol Surg Oncol. 1991;17(10):809–13.
14. Mani R, Margolis DJ, Shukla V, et al. Optimizing technology use for chronic lower-extremity wound healing: a consensus document. Int J Low Extrem Wounds. 2016;15(2):102–19.
15. Erickson CA, Lanza DJ, Karp DL, et al. Healing of venous ulcers in an ambulatory care program: the roles of chronic venous insufficiency and patient compliance. J Vasc Surg. 1995;22(5):629–36.
16. Mayberry JC, Moneta GL, Taylor LM Jr, et al. Fifteen-year results of ambulatory compression therapy for chronic venous ulcers. Surgery. 1991;109(5):575–81.
17. Nelson EA, Bell-Syer SE. Compression for preventing recurrence of venous ulcers. Cochrane Database Syst Rev. 2014;(9):CD002303.
18. Raju S, Hollis K, Neglen P. Use of compression stockings in chronic venous disease: patient compliance and efficacy. Ann Vasc Surg. 2007;21(6):790–5.
19. Van Hecke A, Grypdonck M, Defloor T. A review of why patients with leg ulcers do not adhere to treatment. J Clin Nurs. 2009;18(3):337–49.
20. Weller CD, Buchbinder R, Johnston RV. Interventions for helping people adhere to compression treatments for venous leg ulceration. Cochrane Database Syst Rev. 2016;3:CD008378.
21. Callam MJ, Harper DR, Dale JJ, et al. Arterial disease in chronic leg ulceration: an underestimated hazard? Lothian and Forth Valley leg ulcer study. Br Med J (Clin Res Ed). 1987;294(6577):929–31.
22. Humphreys ML, Stewart AH, Gohel MS, et al. Management of mixed arterial and venous leg ulcers. Br J Surg. 2007;94(9):1104–7.
23. Partsch H, Damstra RJ, Tazelaar DJ, et al. Multicentre, randomised controlled trial of four-layer bandaging versus short-stretch bandaging in the treatment of venous leg ulcers. VASA. 2001;30(2):108–13.
24. Milic DJ, Zivic SS, Bogdanovic DC, et al. Risk factors related to the failure of venous leg ulcers to heal with compression treatment. J Vasc Surg. 2009;49(5):1242–7.
25. Margolis DJ, Berlin JA, Strom BL. Risk factors associated with the failure of a venous leg ulcer to heal. Arch Dermatol. 1999;135(8):920–6.
26. Labropoulos N, Wang ED, Lanier ST, et al. Factors associated with poor healing and recurrence of venous ulceration. Plast Reconstr Surg. 2012;129(1):179–86.
27. Mosti G. Wound care in venous ulcers. Phlebology. 2013;28(Suppl 1):79–85.
28. Raju S, Neglen P. High prevalence of nonthrombotic iliac vein lesions in chronic venous disease: a permissive role in pathogenicity. J Vasc Surg. 2006;44(1):136–43; discussion 44.
29. Neglen P, Thrasher TL, Raju S. Venous outflow obstruction: an underestimated contributor to chronic venous disease. J Vasc Surg. 2003;38(5):879–85.
30. Akesson H, Brudin L, Dahlstrom JA, et al. Venous function assessed during a 5 year period after acute ilio-femoral venous thrombosis treated with anticoagulation. Eur J Vasc Surg. 1990;4(1):43–8.

31. Neglen P, Raju S. Intravascular ultrasound scan evaluation of the obstructed vein. J Vasc Surg. 2002;35(4):694–700.
32. Raju S, Darcey R, Neglen P. Unexpected major role for venous stenting in deep reflux disease. J Vasc Surg. 2010;51(2):401–8; discussion 8.
33. Puggioni A, Kistner RL, Eklof B, et al. Surgical disobliteration of postthrombotic deep veins—endophlebectomy—is feasible. J Vasc Surg. 2004;39(5):1048–52; discussion 52.
34. Shaydakov E, Porembskaya O, Geroulakos G. The May-Husni procedure: a reappraisal. Eur J Vasc Endovasc Surg. 2015;50(4):513–7.
35. Recek C, Pojer H. Ambulatory pressure gradient in the veins of the lower extremity. VASA. 2000;29(3):187–90.
36. Pollack AA, Taylor BE, Myers TT, et al. The effect of exercise and body position on the venous pressure at the ankle in patients having venous valvular defects. J Clin Invest. 1949;28(3):559–63.
37. Mauck KF, Asi N, Undavalli C, et al. Systematic review and meta-analysis of surgical interventions versus conservative therapy for venous ulcers. J Vasc Surg. 2014;60(2 Suppl):60S–70S.e1–2.
38. Papadakis KG, Christopoulos D, Hobbs JT, et al. Descending phlebography in patients with venous ulceration: hemodynamic implications. Int. Angiol. 2015;34(3):263–8.
39. Ting AC, Cheng SW, Wu LL, et al. Changes in venous hemodynamics after superficial vein surgery for mixed superficial and deep venous insufficiency. World J Surg. 2001;25(2):122–5.
40. Raju S, Fredericks RK, Neglen PN, et al. Durability of venous valve reconstruction techniques for "primary" and postthrombotic reflux. J Vasc Surg. 1996;23(2):357–66; discussion 66–7.
41. Kistner RL. Surgical repair of the incompetent femoral vein valve. Arch Surg (Chicago, IL: 1960). 1975;110(11):1336–42.
42. Maleti O, Perrin M. Reconstructive surgery for deep vein reflux in the lower limbs: techniques, results and indications. Eur J Vasc Endovasc Surg. 2011;41(6):837–48.
43. Gohel MS, Barwell JR, Taylor M, et al. Long term results of compression therapy alone versus compression plus surgery in chronic venous ulceration (ESCHAR): randomised controlled trial. BMJ (Clin Res Ed). 2007;335(7610):83.
44. Sinabulya H, Ostmyren R, Blomgren L. Editor's choice—mid-term outcomes of endovenous laser ablation in patients with active and healed venous ulcers: a follow-up study. Eur J Vasc Endovasc Surg. 2017;53(5):710–6.
45. Gohel MS, Heatley F, Liu X, et al. A randomized trial of early endovenous ablation in venous ulceration. N Engl J Med. 2018;378(22):2105–14.
46. Viarengo LM, Poterio-Filho J, Poterio GM, et al. Endovenous laser treatment for varicose veins in patients with active ulcers: measurement of intravenous and perivenous temperatures during the procedure. Dermatol Surg. 2007;33(10):1234–42; discussion 41–2.
47. Alden PB, Lips EM, Zimmerman KP, et al. Chronic venous ulcer: minimally invasive treatment of superficial axial and perforator vein reflux speeds healing and reduces recurrence. Ann Vasc Surg. 2013;27(1):75–83.
48. Raju S, Lurie F, O'Donnell TF Jr. Compression use in the era of endovenous interventions and wound care centers. J Vasc Surg Venous Lymphat Disord. 2016;4(3):346–54.
49. Disselhoff BC, der Kinderen DJ, Kelder JC, et al. Five-year results of a randomized clinical trial comparing endovenous laser ablation with cryostripping for great saphenous varicose veins. Br J Surg. 2011;98(8):1107–11.
50. Siribumrungwong B, Noorit P, Wilasrusmee C, et al. A systematic review and meta-analysis of randomised controlled trials comparing endovenous ablation and surgical intervention in patients with varicose vein. Eur J Vasc Endovasc Surg. 2012;44(2):214–23.
51. Gloviczki P, Comerota AJ, Dalsing MC, et al. The care of patients with varicose veins and associated chronic venous diseases: clinical practice guidelines of the Society for Vascular Surgery and the American Venous Forum. J Vasc Surg. 2011;53(5 Suppl):2s–48s.
52. Joh JH, Kim WS, Jung IM, et al. Consensus for the treatment of varicose vein with radiofrequency ablation. Vasc Specialist Int. 2014;30(4):105–12.

53. Galanopoulos G, Lambidis C. Minimally invasive treatment of varicose veins: endovenous laser ablation (EVLA). Int J Surg (Lond, Engl). 2012;10(3):134–9.
54. Schwarz T, von Hodenberg E, Furtwangler C, et al. Endovenous laser ablation of varicose veins with the 1470-nm diode laser. J Vasc Surg. 2010;51(6):1474–8.
55. van Eekeren RR, Boersma D, de Vries JP, et al. Update of endovenous treatment modalities for insufficient saphenous veins—a review of literature. Semin Vasc Surg. 2014;27(2):118–36.
56. Leung CC, Carradice D, Wallace T, et al. Endovenous laser ablation versus mechanochemical ablation with ClariVein((R)) in the management of superficial venous insufficiency (LAMA trial): study protocol for a randomised controlled trial. Trials. 2016;17(1):421.
57. Whiteley MS, Dos Santos SJ, Lee CT, et al. Mechanochemical ablation causes endothelial and medial damage to the vein wall resulting in deeper penetration of sclerosant compared with sclerotherapy alone in extrafascial great saphenous vein using an ex vivo model. J Vasc Surg Venous Lymphat Disord. 2017;5(3):370–7.
58. Almeida JI, Min RJ, Raabe R, et al. Cyanoacrylate adhesive for the closure of truncal veins: 60-day swine model results. Vasc Endovasc Surg. 2011;45(7):631–5.
59. Whiteley MS. Glue, steam and Clarivein—best practice techniques and evidence. Phlebology. 2015;30(2 Suppl):24–8.
60. Kheirelseid EAH, Crowe G, Sehgal R, et al. Systematic review and meta-analysis of randomized controlled trials evaluating long-term outcomes of endovenous management of lower extremity varicose veins. J Vasc Surg Venous Lymphat Disord. 2018;6(2):256–70.
61. Bacha EA, Chai P, Undar A. Outcomes of the twelfth international conference on pediatric mechanical circulatory support systems and pediatric cardiopulmonary perfusion. Artif Organs. 2017;41(1):7–10.
62. Pannier F, Rabe E, Maurins U. 1470 nm diode laser for endovenous ablation (EVLA) of incompetent saphenous veins—a prospective randomized pilot study comparing warm and cold tumescence anaesthesia. VASA. 2010;39(3):249–55.
63. Vos CG, Unlu C, Bosma J, et al. A systematic review and meta-analysis of two novel techniques of nonthermal endovenous ablation of the great saphenous vein. J Vasc Surg Venous Lymphat Disord. 2017;5(6):880–96.
64. Lane T, Bootun R, Dharmarajah B, et al. A multi-centre randomised controlled trial comparing radiofrequency and mechanical occlusion chemically assisted ablation of varicose veins—final results of the Venefit versus Clarivein for varicose veins trial. Phlebology. 2017;32(2):89–98.
65. Morrison N, Gibson K, McEnroe S, et al. Randomized trial comparing cyanoacrylate embolization and radiofrequency ablation for incompetent great saphenous veins (VeClose). J Vasc Surg. 2015;61(4):985–94.
66. Calcagno D, Rossi JA, Ha C. Effect of saphenous vein diameter on closure rate with ClosureFAST radiofrequency catheter. Vasc Endovasc Surg. 2009;43(6):567–70.
67. Siribumrungwong B, Noorit P, Wilasrusmee C, et al. Cost-utility analysis of great saphenous vein ablation with radiofrequency, foam and surgery in the emerging health-care setting of Thailand. Phlebology. 2016;31(8):573–81.
68. Tellings SS, Ceulen RP, Sommer A. Surgery and endovenous techniques for the treatment of small saphenous varicose veins: a review of the literature. Phlebology. 2011;26(5):179–84.
69. Paravastu SC, Horne M, Dodd PD. Endovenous ablation therapy (laser or radiofrequency) or foam sclerotherapy versus conventional surgical repair for short saphenous varicose veins. Cochrane Database Syst Rev. 2016;11:CD010878.
70. Mosti G, De Maeseneer M, Cavezzi A, et al. Society for Vascular Surgery and American Venous Forum Guidelines on the management of venous leg ulcers: the point of view of the International Union of Phlebology. Int. Angiol. 2015;34(3):202–18.
71. Lawrence PF, Alktaifi A, Rigberg D, et al. Endovenous ablation of incompetent perforating veins is effective treatment for recalcitrant venous ulcers. J Vasc Surg. 2011;54(3):737–42.
72. Kiguchi MM, Hager ES, Winger DG, et al. Factors that influence perforator thrombosis and predict healing with perforator sclerotherapy for venous ulceration without axial reflux. J Vasc Surg. 2014;59(5):1368–76.

73. Masuda EM, Kessler DM, Lurie F, et al. The effect of ultrasound-guided sclerotherapy of incompetent perforator veins on venous clinical severity and disability scores. J Vasc Surg. 2006;43(3):551–6; discussion 6–7.
74. Cronenwett JL, Johnston KW. Rutherford's vascular surgery. Philadelphia, PA: Elsevier; 2014.
75. Katsenis K. Micronized purified flavonoid fraction (MPFF): a review of its pharmacological effects, therapeutic efficacy and benefits in the management of chronic venous insufficiency. Curr Vasc Pharmacol. 2005;3(1):1–9.
76. Smith PC. Daflon 500 mg and venous leg ulcer: new results from a meta-analysis. Angiology. 2005;56(Suppl 1):S33–9.
77. Kakkos S, Nicolaides A. Efficacy of micronized purified flavonoid fraction (Daflon(R)) on improving individual symptoms, signs and quality of life in patients with chronic venous disease: a systematic review and meta-analysis of randomized double-blind placebo-controlled trials. Int Angiol. 2018;37(2):143–54.
78. Wu B, Lu J, Yang M, et al. Sulodexide for treating venous leg ulcers. Cochrane Database Syst Rev. 2016;(6):CD010694.
79. Pascarella L, Shortell CK. Medical management of venous ulcers. Semin Vasc Surg. 2015;28(1):21–8.
80. Jull AB, Arroll B, Parag V, et al. Pentoxifylline for treating venous leg ulcers. Cochrane Database Syst Rev. 2012;12:CD001733.
81. Ye J, Mani R. A systematic review and meta-analysis of nutritional supplementation in chronic lower extremity wounds. Int J Low Extrem Wounds. 2016;15(4):296–302.
82. de Oliveira Carvalho PE, Magolbo NG, De Aquino RF, et al. Oral aspirin for treating venous leg ulcers. Cochrane Database Syst Rev. 2016;2:CD009432.
83. Jull A, Wadham A, Bullen C, et al. Low dose aspirin as adjuvant treatment for venous leg ulceration: pragmatic, randomised, double blind, placebo controlled trial (Aspirin4VLU). BMJ (Clin Res Ed). 2017;359:j5157.
84. Brown A. Life-style advice and self-care strategies for venous leg ulcer patients: what is the evidence? J Wound Care. 2012;21(7):342–4, 6, 8–50.
85. Smith D, Lane R, McGinnes R, et al. What is the effect of exercise on wound healing in patients with venous leg ulcers? A systematic review. Int Wound J. 2018;15(3):441–53.
86. Davies JA, Bull RH, Farrelly IJ, et al. A home-based exercise programme improves ankle range of motion in long-term venous ulcer patients. Phlebology. 2007;22(2):86–9.
87. Padberg FT Jr, Johnston MV, Sisto SA. Structured exercise improves calf muscle pump function in chronic venous insufficiency: a randomized trial. J Vasc Surg. 2004;39(1):79–87.
88. Jull A, Parag V, Walker N, et al. The prepare pilot RCT of home-based progressive resistance exercises for venous leg ulcers. J Wound Care. 2009;18(12):497–503.
89. Kelechi TJ, Green A, Dumas B, et al. Online coaching for a lower limb physical activity program for individuals at home with a history of venous ulcers. Home Healthc Nurse. 2010;28(10):596–605.
90. Alavi A, Sibbald RG, Phillips TJ, et al. What's new: management of venous leg ulcers: treating venous leg ulcers. J Am Acad Dermatol. 2016;74(4):643–64; quiz 65–6.
91. Serra R, Rizzuto A, Rossi A, et al. Skin grafting for the treatment of chronic leg ulcers—a systematic review in evidence-based medicine. Int Wound J. 2017;14(1):149–57.
92. Barber C, Watt A, Pham C, et al. Influence of bioengineered skin substitutes on diabetic foot ulcer and venous leg ulcer outcomes. J Wound Care. 2008;17(12):517–27.
93. Barnes MD, Mani R, Barretr DF, White JE. Changes in skin microcirculation at periulcerous sites in patients with chronic venous ulcers during leg elevation. Phlebology. 1992;7:36–9.
94. Barnes MD, Mani R, Barretr DF, White JE. How to measure changes in oedema in patients with chronic venous ulcers? Phlebology. 1992;7:31–5.
95. Davies HO, Popplewell M, Singhal R, et al. Obesity and lower limb venous disease—the epidemic of phlebesity. Phlebology. 2017;32(4):227–33.
96. Musil D, Kaletova M, Herman J. Age, body mass index and severity of primary chronic venous disease. Biomed Papers Med Fac Univ Palacky Olomouc Czechoslovakia. 2011;155(4):367–71.
97. van Rij AM, De Alwis CS, Jiang P, et al. Obesity and impaired venous function. Eur J Vasc Endovasc Surg. 2008;35(6):739–44.

Chapter 6
The Use of Compression to Treat Venous Leg Ulcers: The Inadequacy of Current Compression Systems Especially in Tropical Nations

Harikrishna K. R. Nair

Abstract Venous leg ulcers are a chronic problem and the mainstay of treatment is compression bandaging. There are many systems of compression bandaging which include short stretch and four-layer bandaging. However, there is always a problem in these systems when it comes to the usage in tropical nations due to the prevalent heat and the humidity. Level of activity plays an important role. Therefore, the health care professional has to have the knowledge and the training to do it well so there is graduated pressure during static and dynamic activity. In addition, the patients have to be engaged and informed about the compression bandaging system so that they don't remove it. This is crucial for the management of the venous ulcer. A proper system has to be used to allow venous return and manage the ulcer comprehensively. Proper dressings are also needed according to the wound bed, edge and the peri-wound skin.

Keywords Venous ulcer · Compression bandaging · Tropical nations · Knowledge · Training · Compliance · Dressing

6.1 Introduction

Leg ulcers are very common type of wounds occurring in many countries and there are many causes such as chronic venous insufficiency, arterial disease, mixed, diabetes, lymphoedema, trauma and malignancy. Venous ulcers due to chronic venous insufficiency are the commonest leg ulcers.

H. K. R. Nair (✉)
Wound Care Unit, Department of Internal Medicine, Kuala Lumpur Hospital, Kuala Lumpur, Malaysia

Department of Surgery, Institute of Medical Sciences, Banares Hindu University, Varanasi, Uttar Pradesh, India

R. Mani et al. (eds.), *Compression and Chronic Wound Management*, https://doi.org/10.1007/978-3-030-01195-6_6

Many of these ulcers are chronic and are stuck in the inflammatory phase with elevated protease activity. The mainstay of management involves the utilization of compression bandaging [1]. There are various compression bandaging systems such as the single layer, double and four layer. The four layer bandaging system is the gold standard. Randomized Control Trials in the Cochrane Review by O'Meara S showed that the four-layer bandaging was effective in treating venous ulcers [2]. The standard method in the UK comprises Orthopaedic wool, Crepe bandage, Elastic bandage and Cohesive retaining layer. However, nowadays the four layer compression system is used for patients who are not active or ambulating while the two layer systems are used for active mobile patients. Lazareth et al. [3] noted that the two layer system was not seen to be any less effective than a well-known four layer bandaging system in the management of VLUs. Furthermore, the two layer bandaging system was considered to be easier to apply, representing an alternative to the conventional treatment with four layer bandaging currently available [4]. The compression bandaging systems have different graduated pressure gradients to help with the venous return and reduce the oedema. The pressure has to be sufficient to exert its effect during resting and movement whereby the resting and dynamic pressure should be measured with a suitable pressure gauge.

Training in using compression with a proper technique and giving sufficient pressure is crucial. Many health care professionals have insufficient knowledge and hands on training. However, our experience is that often patients remove the compression bandaging and are not compliant to treatment protocols due the fact that it is very uncomfortable to use.

In general, the failures of compression therapy are not caused by poor compression material but due to poor knowledge and application techniques of the care providers.

In addition, the weather is a huge problem in tropical countries. The hot and humid weather contributes to the lack of compliance in these groups of patients. It is truly uncomfortable. Therefore, new systems which are efficacious and are comfortable to be utilized are important. Most systems were designed to be used in Caucasians in cold climates which is a complete contrast to patients in the tropics. Short stretch bandages are now commonly used especially in the tropical countries. Moody in 1999 did a study comparing the short stretch bandage and the long stretch bandage in 52 patients with venous ulcers and noted that there was more reduction in the wound bed size in the short stretch group.

Some countries actually modify the system by using orthopaedic wool and cohesive bandages conforming to the dictum that any pressure is better than no pressure at all. In addition, there is the factor of cost which inhibits some clinicians in getting the readily available short stretch bandages commercially.

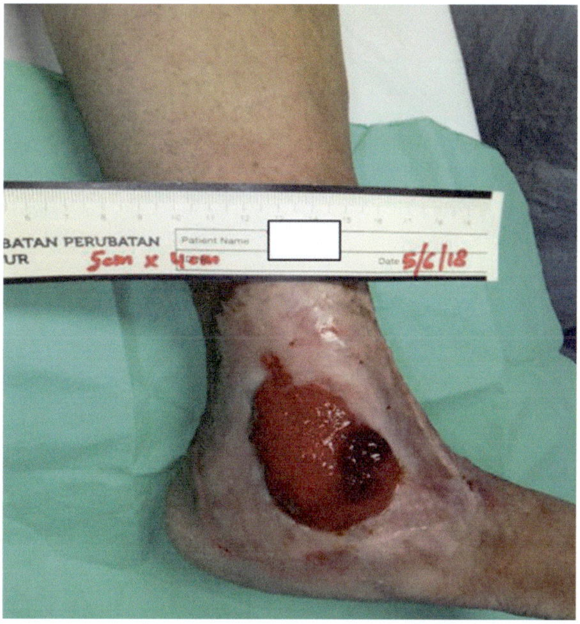

Picture 6.1 Chronic venous ulcer at the gaiter region of the left leg

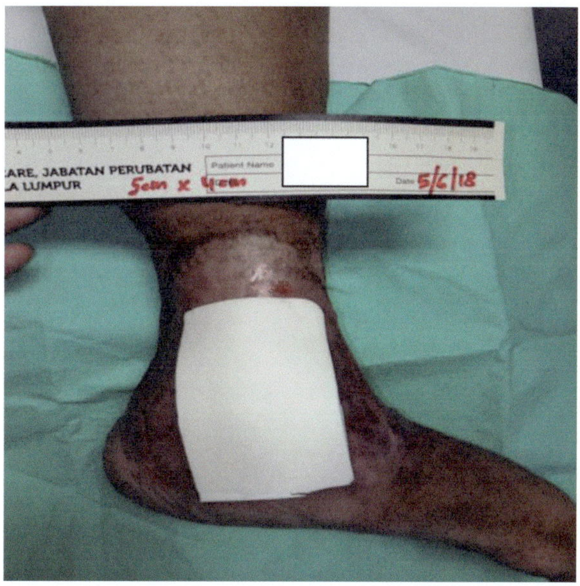

Picture 6.2 Dressing with tender lipido colloid and nano oligosaccharide factor foam dressing

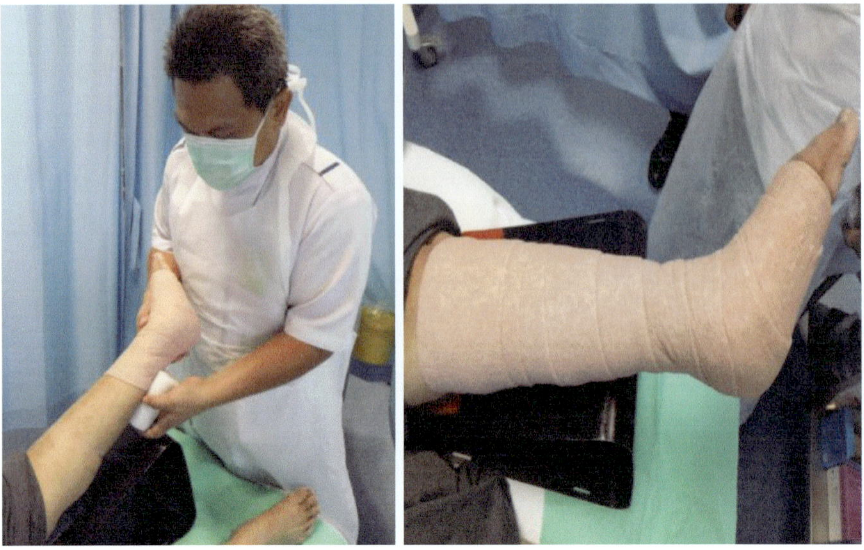

Picture 6.3 First layer bandaging—using the Sigg technique (figure of 8)

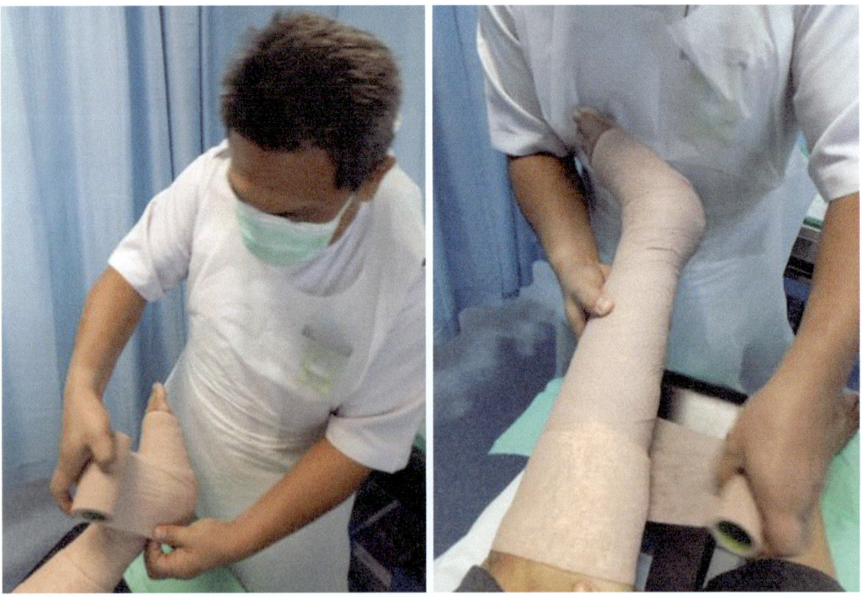

Picture 6.4 Second layer of the two layer system compression bandaging

6.2 Application of a Two Layer Compression Bandage

There are many factors that you have to note and this is shown in Fig. 6.1 from Mazzei et al. [5] which includes slippage, loss of sensitivity, rolling, feeling hot, itching, feeling tightness and exudates in the bandage (Fig. 6.2).

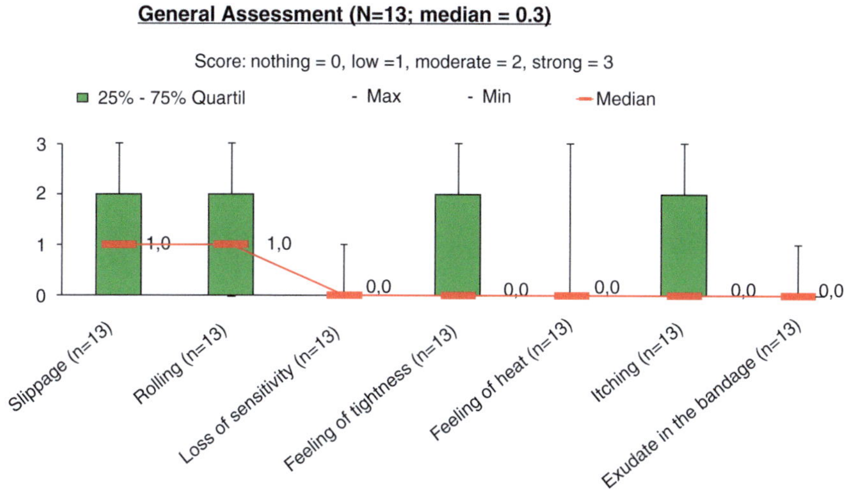

Fig. 6.1 Mazzei et al. [5]: Results of an observation study on thirteen mixed or arterial leg ulcer patients with a new two component system (TCS)

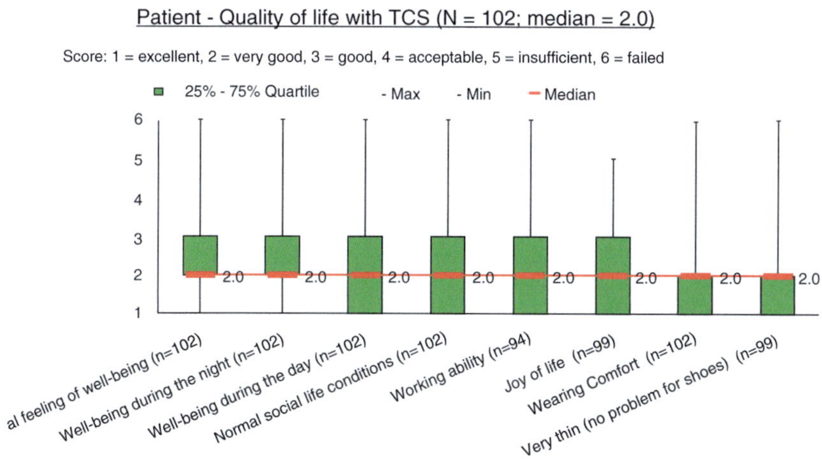

Fig. 6.2 Patients quality of life with TCS (Mazzei et al. [5, 6])

The technical assessment is also very important whereby we have to ask ourselves is it easy to use, thin and no problem for shoes or footwear, comfort and there is sufficient movement of the ankle joint. These are factors that have an impact on patients who are mobile.

6.3 Clinical Cases with the Two Layer Compression Systems

These cases were due to chronic venous insufficiency. The assessment was done using the TIME concept. The wounds were cleansed and bedside sharp debridement was performed. The wounds were dressed with advanced dressings and a two layer compression bandage was applied.

6.4 Case 1

A 56 year old Malay lady developed a wound on the right leg associated with chronic venous insufficiency. She sought treatment from the Dermatology Department, Hospital Kuala Lumpur. On assessment patient had a chronic right leg anterior tibial ulcer with granulation tissue and we suspected that there was a thick layer of biofilm with moderate yellowish exudate and maceration at the periwound area. Patient complaints of localized pain at the wound area. The pain score was 3/10 according to the Visual Analog Score.

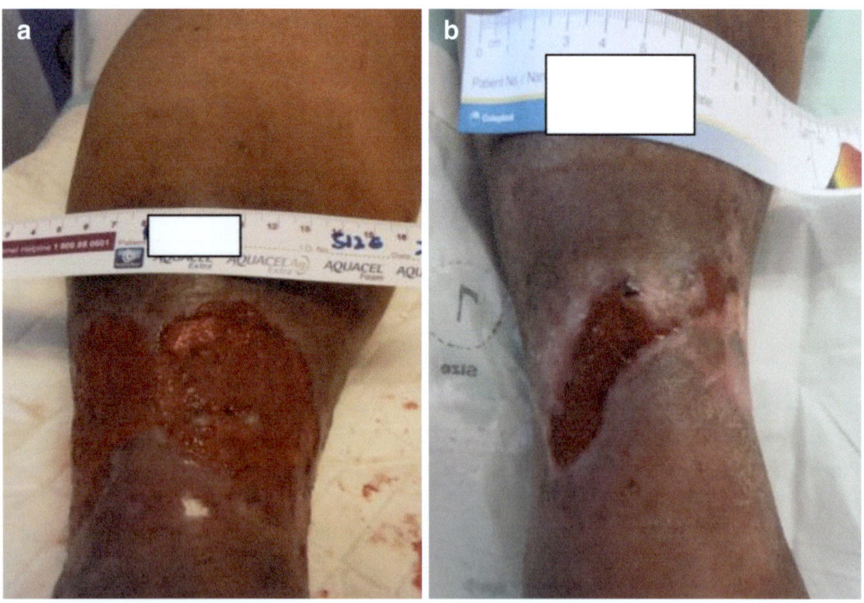

Picture 6.5 (**a**) First week (18 × 7 cm). (**b**) Third week (5 × 2 cm)

6.5 Case 2

A 63 years old Malay gentleman with Type 2 Diabetes Mellitus on Oral Hypoglycaemic Agents presented with a venous ulcer on the right medial malleolus. On assessment the wound was sloughy with biofilm, heavy yellowish exudate, and mild epithelization surrounding the ulcer.

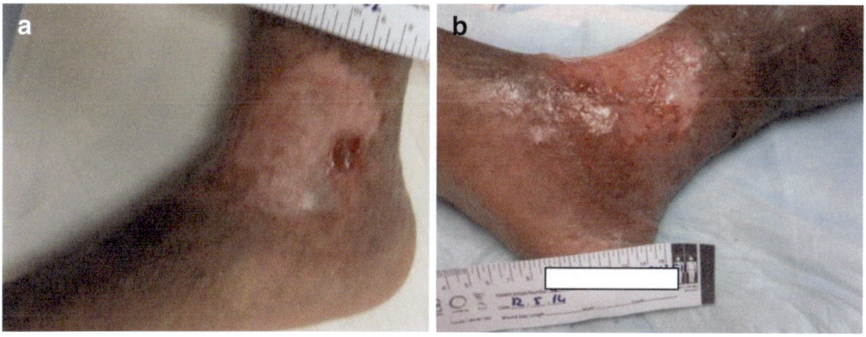

Picture 6.6 (**a**) First week (1 × 1 cm). (**b**) Sixth week (healed)

6.6 Case 3

A 68 year old Malay gentleman with Type 2 Diabetes Mellitus on Oral Hypoglycaemic Agent was seen in the Wound Clinic with a venous ulcer at the left anterior tibial area of the lower limb. On assessment the ulcer had granulation tissue, mild biofilm, moderate yellowish exudate and epithelial tissue surrounding the ulcer.

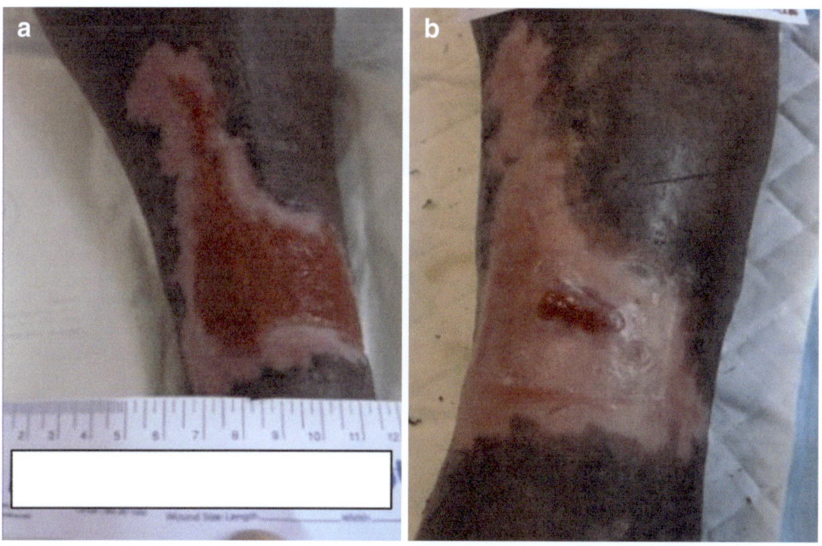

Picture 6.7 (**a**) First week (11 × 7 cm). (**b**) Sixth week (0.5 × 1.5 cm)

6.7 Dressings and Other Modalities

Various dressings have been used to manage venous ulcers such as polyurethane foams, hydrofiber, durafiber and others to manage exudates while anti inflammatory dressings such as collagen, TLC-NOSF and others have been used to manage the inflammation where there is elevated protease activity. New modalities are also available such as topical oxygen therapy which are part of the armamentarium to manage the chronic venous ulcers comprehensively.

The choice of the dressing depends on the condition of the wound bed, the edge and the peri-wound skin. A few cases were showcased here but it is not exhaustive. The dressings are equally important with the choice of compression bandaging because they are the mainstay of management and compliance is a crucial factor. These dressings and compression systems can be removed and this is not good as patient tends to remove them if it is not comfortable or applicable in their daily activities. This conforms to the basic principle that we have to consider the factors that are affecting the patient, changes in the environment and the effect of the caregiver.

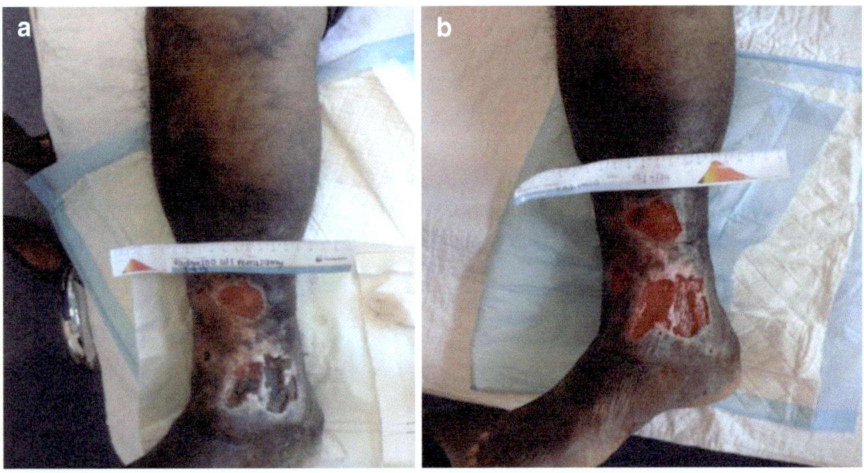

Picture 6.8 (**a**, **b**) Utilization of honey dressing for enzymatic debridement [7]

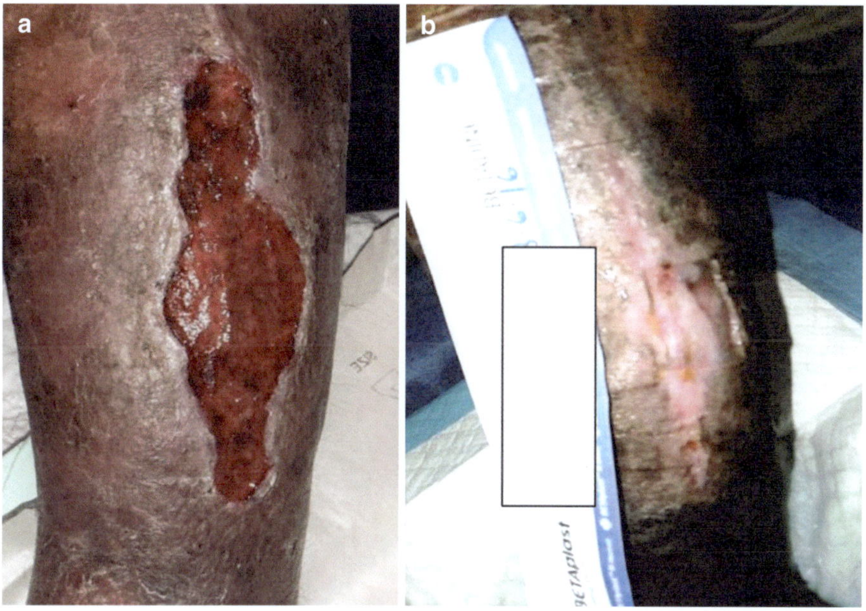

Picture 6.9 (**a**, **b**) Usage of retrotech dressing which consists of gentian violet, surfactant, silver, methylene bluc and polyurethane foam [7]

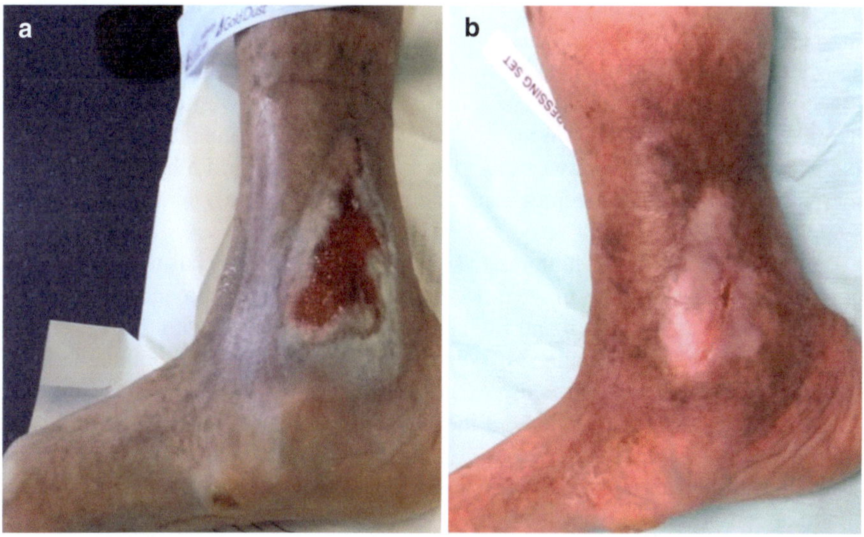

Picture 6.10 (**a**, **b**) Usage of modified collagen and glycerine [7]

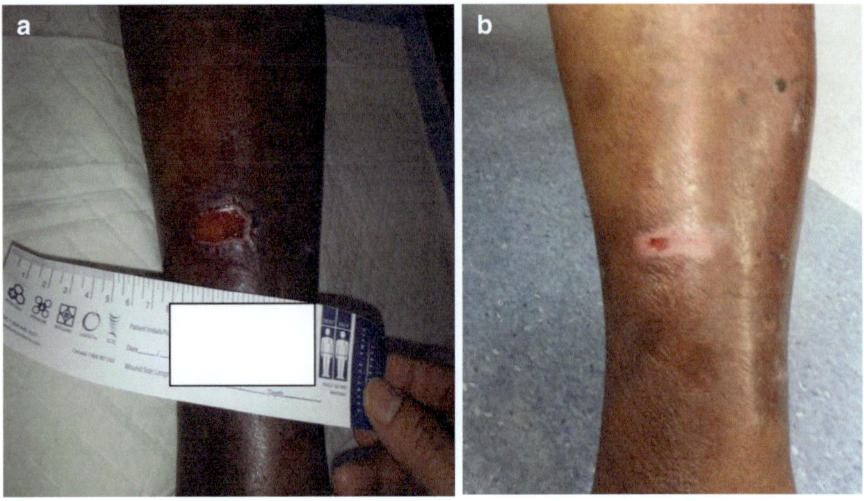

Picture 6.11 (**a**, **b**) Utilization of polyurethane foam with smart pore technology

6.8 Conclusion

In venous ulcers, compression bandaging is the mainstay of treatment [8]. We have to have the proper succinct knowledge and training to be able to apply the bandaging system correctly so that there is sufficient graduated static and dynamic pressure. In addition, the compression system has to be applicable and advantageous especially when it comes to patient compliance. It has to be comfortable in hot and humid conditions especially in the tropical nations so that patients don't remove it. Patients also wear footwear when they go to work and perform other activities and therefore they require a compression system which allows this and alleviates their symptoms.

Patients' lifestyle and health related quality of life (HRQol) has to be taken into consideration and factored in when we plan a management approach with our clients. They have to be in on it and we have to work collectively with the patient and the caregiver. The individualized patient centric management is important and as a clinician we have to look into this. We have to engage the patient and the caregiver in their management and give them the pros and cons of using compression bandaging. Once the ulcer heals, we have to inform them to use compression stockings which is another difficult part. Nelson EA noted that there is evidence from one trial that compression hosiery reduces rates of re-ulceration of venous ulcers compared with no compression [9]. Of course, surgery and other treatment methods exist and are presented in other chapters in this book. In all these cases, subsequently, these patients have to be on compression. Short stretch bandages are the most commonly used.

References

1. Partsch H, Mortimer P. Compression for leg wounds. Br J Dermatol. 2015;173:359–69.
2. O'Meara S, Cullum N, Nelson EA, Dunville JC. Compression for venous leg ulcers. Cochrane Database Systemic Review. 2013;11:CD000265. https://doi.org/10.1002/14651858.CD000265.pub3.
3. Lazareth I, Moffatt C, Dissemond J, Lesne Padieu AS, Truchetet F, Beissert S, Wicks G, Tilbe H, Sauvadet A, Bohbot S, Meaume S. Efficacy of two compression system in the management of VLUs: Results of a European RCT. J Wound Care. 2012;21:11.
4. Moody M. Comparison of Rosidal K and Surepress in the treatment of venous ulcers. Br J Nurs. 1999;8(6):345–55.
5. Mazzei S, Mosti G, Collarte A, Dini V, Bahr S, Coulborne A, Hampel Kalthoff C, Zell C, Brambilla R, Abel M. Results of an observation study on thirteen mixed or arterial leg ulcer patients with a new two-component-system (TCS): EWMA 15-17, Copenhagen, Denmark (ID:47688); 2013.
6. Mazzei S, Mosti G, Collarte A, Dini V, Bahr S, Coulborne A, Hampel Kalthoff C, Zell C, Brambilla R, Abel M. Results of an observational study on 102 leg ulcer patients with a new two-component-system.
7. Nair HKR. Compendium of wound care dressing. 4th edn; 2017.
8. Manual of wound care. Malaysia: Ministry of Health; 2014.
9. Nelson EA, Bell-Syer SEM. Compression for preventing recurrence of venous ulcers. Cochrane Database Syst Rev. 2014;9:CD002303. https://doi.org/10.1002/14651858.CD002303.pub3.

Chapter 7
The Use of Compression to Treat Venous Leg Ulcers in Traditional Chinese Medicine Practice

Xian Xiao, Qi Wang, Yao Huang, Pengwen Ni, Yunfei Wang, and Ting Xie

Abstract Venous leg ulcers are common in China where both Western (Allopathic) and Traditional Chinese Medicine systems coexist. This chapter is focused on the TCM and the use of compression and other techniques to manage this condition. The report is based on translation of reports in Chinese language and give the reader an understanding of the use of oral and topical medicines and the use of compression in modern China where up to date modern diagnostic facilities exist in both systems of care.

Keywords Venous leg ulcers · Traditional Chinese medicine (TCM) · Compression

Elasticated compression has been advocated and is used in case of venous leg ulcers (VLU) in the absence of peripheral arterial disease (PAD), together with wound care [1]. Compression is considered to be a key element for therapy as prevention for VLU since compression can deliver external pressure against unrelieved or ambulatory venous hypertension, which is regarded the core factor of the pathogenesis of VLU [2]. For these reasons, compression is accepted as an important means for wound management of VLU. In China two systems of medicine are practiced: Western (or Allopathic) medicine as well as Traditional Chinese Medicine (TCM) coexist. Patients chose the system of care in which their condition should be managed: some clinicians trained in the Western (or Allopathic) system of medicine are also accredited to prescribe TCM medicines. On the other hand, TCM hospitals are often major facilities with all the latest diagnostic imaging techniques staffed by highly trained clinicians, many with post graduate qualifications. The central aim of this book is to discuss compression with evidence of its use as well as limitations,

X. Xiao · Q. Wang · Y. Huang · P. Ni · T. Xie (✉)
Wound Healing Center at Emergency Department, Ninth People's Hospital, Shanghai Jiao Tong University School of Medicine, Shanghai, China

Y. Wang
LongHua Hospital, Shanghai University of Traditional Chinese Medicine, Shanghai, China

R. Mani et al. (eds.), *Compression and Chronic Wound Management*,
https://doi.org/10.1007/978-3-030-01195-6_7

the role of surgery as well as recently innovated devices that offer compression. This chapter will draw attention to the role of TCM in this context.

Traditional Chinese Medicine (TCM) has a thousand years of history of treating wound diseases. Some important records exist of work done 500 hundred years ago. Currently a number of reports exist addressing the application of TCM to treat wounds. Accessing this literature for readers whose first language is English is no mean task. TCM literature on treating wounds is in Chinese, some of it 'medical' ancient Chinese as found when it was sought to check discussion of compression use in TCM. However, the authors have done their best to interpret some reports to the readers in the sincere belief that would be helpful to understand compression in TCM.

Compendium of Materia Medica (Ben Cao Gang Mu), a great work written by Li Shizhen, a famous medical scientist in the Ming Dynasty (A.D. 1552), is the "Bible" of TCM [3]. The book has almost two million Chinese characters, listing 1892 kinds of medical substances. The English version of the book was published in 2003. In this book, a word "Lian Chuang" was used which refers to leg ulcers, and most part of them is VLU [4]. Li Shizhen recorded a couple of methods including oral and external/topical treatments of leg ulcers in the TCM system of care. For VLU, within total 33 kinds of prescription of external treatment, two of them were about compression (the ancient Chinese name was "Chan Fu") [5]. From here we got to know that, the ancient medical scientist of China had realized the importance of compression when treating leg ulcers, even though they may or not know about venous hypertension.

For the method of compression in TCM, a few reports describe the details of compression therapy. In most general hospitals, especially within tertiary care, multi-layered garments or at least single layer elastic bandage must be applied, while in TCM, compression is often employed combined with topical use of TCM ointment or paste. This is not far from practice outside China be it in the West or within Asia.

Usually, the topical used TCM medications with the function of debridement or promoting granulation is applied depending on the status of the wound, and a single layer of gauze or cotton pad is used to cover the wound. This is followed by an elastic bandage which is wrapped around the lower leg. The results showed the improvement of wound bed preparation and wound healing.

In some other reports, a combination of TCM lotion, TCM ointment, and compression were highly regarded as efficacious for treating VLU [6]. As the first step, TCM lotion was used to wash the wound bed and reach the effect of cleansing, antibacteria and to improve the microcirculation. (Fig. 7.1) After that, TCM ointment (Fig. 7.2) and compression (Fig. 7.3) were used in that order.

Basically, it is very difficult to find a complete correspondence when we are going to translate the whole profile of TCM to the audience from English speaking countries, on account of the very different philosophy of TCM. In the TCM system, the assessment of VLU is expressed as deficiency-excess and yin-yang balance. Based on the result of TCM assessment, the prescription of TCM is selected and determined for topical use. To simplify matters for readers equivalence of TCM in

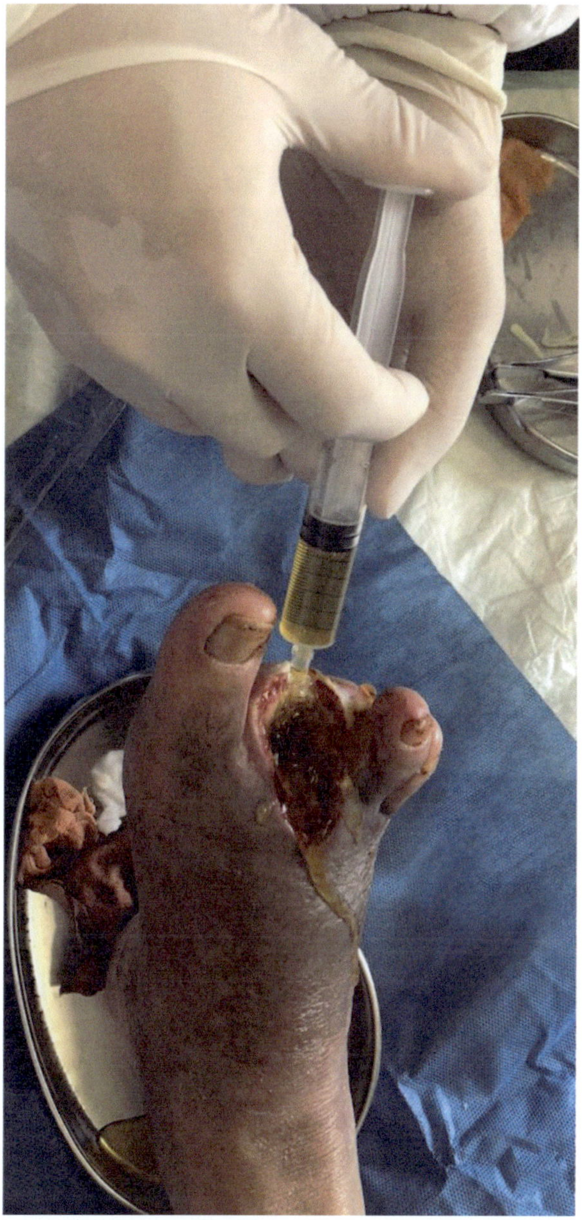

Fig. 7.1 Wound cleansing in foot ulcer with TCM lotion

the context of VLU treatment may be considered as TCM lotion as saline and TCM ointment as advanced dressings. External compression using garments follow this.

More pleasingly, there is a trend to integrate traditional Chinese and western medicine. In the past decades, TCM methods have been used in many wound healing centers in general hospitals, and modern medical diagnostic and therapeutic

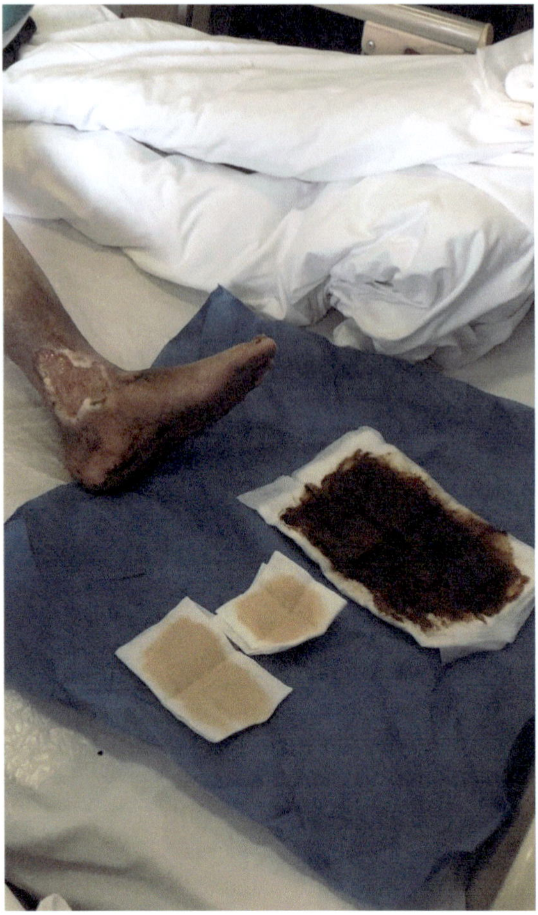

Fig. 7.2 TCM ointment was coated in a layer of gauze and used topically over the wound size

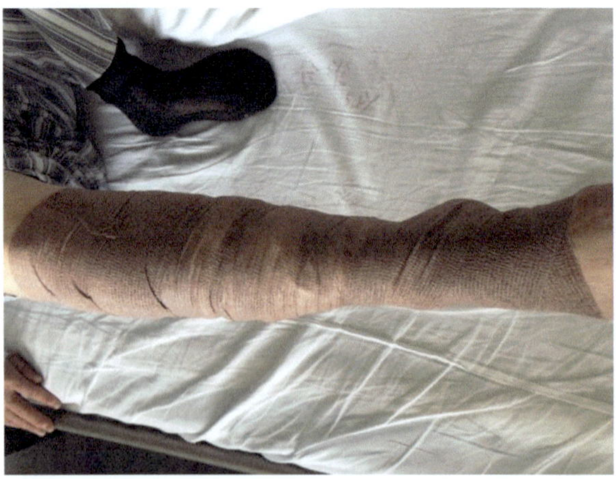

Fig. 7.3 Elastic compression was applied wrapping the lower leg

methods have also been engaged in TCM hospitals. X ray, CT, MRI, ultrasound Doppler, et al., provide information of assessment of wound diseases, while surgery, negative pressure wound therapy and other adjuvants are also used to treat wounds in TCM hospitals. For compression, it has been widely accepted in most Tertiary TCM Hospitals.

Considering the long history and wide use of TCM, it must be realized that, the research papers with TCM published in international journals, not only on compression, but also on other aspects of wound diseases, have been comparatively not many. Besides the more great effort on clinical research, how to cross the chasm of two different philosophies is a big challenge to national and international colleagues.

Acknowledgments The authors acknowledge Prof. Raj Mani for critical modification to the article.

Authors' contribution: Xian Xiao and Qi Wang administered reviewing literatures. Yao Huang and Pengwen Ni performed translational work. Yunfei Wang provided TCM methods of treating leg ulcers. Ting Xie was responsible to supervising the work and drafting manuscript.

References

1. Mani R, Margolis DJ, Shukla VK, et al. Optimal use of technology to manage chronic lower extremity wounds: a consensus document. Int J Low Extrem Wounds. 2016;15(2):102–19.
2. Xie T, Ye J, Rerkasem K, Mani R. The venous ulcer continues to be a clinical challenge: an update. Burns Trauma. 2018;15:6–18.
3. Li S, Luo X. Compendium of Materia Medica. China: Foreign Languages Press; 2003.
4. Chen H, Liu M. Prescription in compendium of materia medica treating leg ulcers and its modern research. LISHIZHEN Med Mater Med Res. 2001;12(2):173.
5. Wang W, Zhu C, Xu Q, Liu T, Zhang C. The research on external therapy of leg ulcers. J External Ther TCM. 2017;26(2):46–8.
6. Zhang Y, Wang X, Li W, Wang Y. Observation of the effect of herbal fumigation and washout with Qingyingfang plus topical medicated bandaging on ecthyma. Mod J Int Tradit Chin West Med. 2012;21(1):6–8.

Chapter 8
Compression Therapy in Lymphoedema

V. K. Shukla and Vivek Srivastava

Abstract Lymphoedema is a distressing condition due to accumulation of excess of lymph into intertstitial space causing not only unsightly swelling but also its complications of skin and psychological adverse effects. Lymphoedema may be primary, as a result of a genetic abnormality, or secondary, as a result of injury, including non-accidental injury, or following treatments such as radiotherapy and/or surgery. Compression therapy is the mainstay of lymphoedema management as this condition is rarely curable and has high chances of relapse. Thus selection of appropriate compression therapy both for the amelioration of acute condition and maintenance of remission is needed. The specific indications of the type of compression required and its specific contraindication for use must be kept in mind so that treatment adherence can be ensured.

Keywords Lymphoedema · Compression · Bandage · Garments · Evidence

8.1 Introduction

It's an irony that although breast cancer related lymphoedema was described almost a century back the lymphatic system and its pathologies have been the subject of passive neglect till late [1]. Lymphoedema is described as the swelling of any part of the body due to inefficient lymphatic system and eventual thickening of skin and soft tissue. By and large lymphoedema remains an incurable disease till date.

V. K. Shukla · V. Srivastava (✉)
Department of General Surgery, Institute of Medical Sciences, Banaras Hindu University, Varanasi, Uttar Pradesh, India

R. Mani et al. (eds.), *Compression and Chronic Wound Management*,
https://doi.org/10.1007/978-3-030-01195-6_8

8.2 Pathophysiology

Lymphoedema is a protein rich fluid accumulation in the interstitium as a result of net excess filtration of fluid from the arterial end of capillary to the venular end. Various complex and interrelated pressure gradients and mechanical forces result in net accumulation of lymph in the interstitial space [2]. Apart from the changes in pressure and mechanical forces any disruption in lymphatic vessel also leads to accumulation of lymph [3–6].

As a result of this interstitial fluid accumulation there sets in a chronic inflammatory response leading to fibrosis of lymphatic wall and subsequent incompetence [2]. There also occurs concomitant fat deposition and subcutaneous fibrosis over period of time [7–10]. This lipogenesis and fat deposition is the result of transformation of monocytes to adipocytes [11–15]. Research has shown that the chronic inflammation leads to up regulation of fat differentiation markers as well as adipogenic differentiation of stem cells.

8.3 Classification

- Primary Lymphoedema: Lymphoedema occurring as a result of genetic or developmental abnormality of lymphatics. It has a varied presentation from birth (congenital) to puberty (praecox) or even in adults up to 35 years age (tarda)
- Secondary Lymphoedema: Lymphoedema occurring due to disruption or obstruction of normal lymphatics. The damage could be a result of cancer infiltration, inflammatory process resulting from elephantiasis or due to trauma.

8.4 Epidemiology

Lymphoedema is not a very uncommon disease with majority of patients resulting from secondary cause. In developed countries cancer related lymphoedema is the most common etiology contrary to developing country where inflammatory cause supersedes all [16–20]. In tropical countries Filariasis caused by parasitic nimatode Waucheria Bancrofti remains the leading cause. The adult worm lodged in the lymphatic system initiates an inflammatory response leading to vessel hyperplasia and fibrosis. Almost 120 million people in tropics are affected by this disease [21].

8.5 Diagnostic Criteria

The diagnosis of lymphoedema remains clinical primarily with a 10% difference in limb volume taken as cut off to label the disease. Volume measurement can be done using sequential circumference measurement and/or by means of water displacement techniques [22].

Investigations to establish lymphoedema are not a standard requirement, yet among the common ones are Lymphoscintigraphy, CT Scan, MRI or Ultrasound. Measurement of local tissue water can be done by recent methods which include Tissue Dielectric Constant (TDC) or Bio Impedance Spectroscopy (BIS) [23, 24]. Indo Cyanine Green (ICG) lymphoscintigraphy is also a promising tool utilized to detect the abnormality of lymph flow [25].

8.6 Differential Diagnosis

Both unilateral and bilateral limb edema can be caused by diseases other than lymphoedema. This fact demands cautious detection of specific cause so that adequate treatment could be offered. The common reasons for bilateral edema could be congestive heart failure, renal or hepatic insufficiency, hypothyroidism, hypoproteinemia, medication, chronic venous insufficiency or lipidemia [26–28].

Unilateral swelling could be because of Deep Vein thrombosis or post thrombotic limb, arthritis, Baker's cyst or malignancy [29, 30].

8.7 Staging

Lymph edema staging is done by the international society of Lymphology as [31]:

Stage 0—Subclinical stage where swelling is not evident in spite of impaired lymph transport.

Stage 1—Accumulation of fluid that subsides on limb elevation.

Stage 2—Limb elevation alone rarely reduces limb swelling. Edema may or may not be pitting.

Stage 3—Tissue becomes hard and fibrotic with secondary skin charges like thickening, hyperpigmentation, increased skin folds, fat deposition or warty overgrowth.

Unilateral limb lymphoedema severity can be classified based on the difference in limb volume from the unaffected side. It could be mild (>5% to <20% excess limb volume), moderate (20–40% excess limb volume) or severe (>40% excess limb volume).

8.8 Management of Patients with Lymphoedema and Role of Compression

Lymphoedema requires long-term management through co-ordinated care appropriate to the needs of the patients. Care needed for management comes not only from patients but also from care givers and family members so as to improve concordance with treatment regimens and improve quality of life. The treatment for lymphoedema includes a myriad of options including skin care, exercise, manual lymphatic drainage (a form of massage), compression therapy, pneumatic sequential pump therapy, and therapies involving laser treatment and deep oscillation.

Appropriate skin care is essential since it reduces the risk of infections, such as cellulitis. The combination of skin care, exercise, manual lymphatic drainage and compression therapy is often termed decongestive lymphatic therapy [32]. Compression therapy is the most important component of this.

Treatment of lymphoedema tends to be offered in specialist clinics. While these clinics have more recently adopted a skill mix of healthcare professionals, there is still a general consensus that some aspects of treatment should be a feature of the specialist's role. Lymphoedema compression bandaging (LCB) is one such treatment that requires healthcare professionals to undertake further training.

Compression causes an increase in tissue pressure, resulting in the movement or contraction of the anchoring filaments attached to the openings of the lymphatic capillaries. This causes them to open and fill with fluid (lymph). Backflow of fluid in the lymphatics is prevented by valves. When fluid is present in the lymphatic collectors, its propulsion is assisted by rhythmic contractions of muscles during exercise [33]. When the lymphatic system is damaged, compression and exercise increase activity in damaged lymphatics, maximising lymph drainage and reducing oedema [34, 35].

Patients with lymphoedema may present with altered limb shape and deformity because of the distribution of oedema, fat and fibrosclerotic tissue. Compression therapy can be used as an intensive treatment for lymphoedema, reducing limb size and reshaping distortion. It can also be used as a maintenance treatment to prevent progression of symptoms. The International Lymphoedema Framework [36] updated best practice guidelines to include compression as a fundamental component in the treatment of lymphoedema.

Patients undergoing intensive treatment for lymphoedema should be physically and emotionally able to undertake daily intensive therapy, including participation in exercise programs. The level of compression used is determined by daily evaluation of limb volume reduction—high levels of compression are usual. If the patient has difficulty tolerating high levels of compression, the healthcare professional will discontinue intensive therapy and propose an adapted regimen. Intensive therapy usually lasts between 1 and 4 weeks; during this time, treatment is evaluated continuously and appropriate alterations are made according to the patient's needs and the effectiveness of the regimen.

8.9 Sub-bandage Pressures

The efficacy of LCB is determined by the amount of pressure under the bandage (subbandage pressure). The sub-bandage pressure is influenced by the resting pressure, working pressure, elasticity of the application and the pressure at which it is applied.

8.10 Resting and Working Pressure

The short-stretch bandages which are commonly used in LCB have low extensibility. They exert high working pressure and low resting pressure. Resting pressure is the constant pressure externally applied by the bandage. Working pressure is temporary pressure that is generated internally in the muscle and that also affects the deeper tissues. The advantage of using bandages with high working and low resting pressures is that they are usually well tolerated by the wearer. When compared with long-stretch bandaging, relatively higher working pressures are produced by short-stretch bandaging during muscle contraction. These forces are transmitted into the limb to soften fibrotic tissue and facilitate movement of fluid. The relatively lower resting pressure of short-stretch bandages, when compared with long-stretch bandages improves tolerance of compression and helps to minimise circulatory compromise.

8.11 Bandage Elasticity

The static stiffness index (SSI) of a bandage describes its resistance to the deformation caused by a change in limb circumference [18]. The SSI explains the performance of a bandage when transitioning between supine (resting) and standing (working) positions. When a limb changes circumference moving from supine to standing position, a bandage with high SSI will resist deformation and will maintain its original shape. The higher the SSI of a bandage, the greater the pressure increase exerted upon the limb when standing. In general, compression materials that have a high SSI combine high working pressure during standing and walking with a relatively low and tolerable resting pressure when lying [19]. Pascal's law explains how a bandage with a high SSI applies pressure to a limb.

Pascal's law states that, when there is an increase in pressure at any point in a contained fluid, there is an equal increase at every other point in the container. In other words, in a compression system with a high SSI the movement of muscles creates pressure that is evenly distributed throughout the area of the limb under compression. The SSI of a bandage system can be described using the PLACE system:

- **P**ressure equals
- **LA**yers of the bandage applied
- **C**omponents of the bandage system—this factor considers the functions of different
- materials e.g. padding, protection and spot pressure.
- **E**lastic properties—this describes the effect of all combined materials on the resting and working pressures.

The elastic properties of a bandage system can be affected by many factors. If multiple layers of materials are used, the friction between the layers will result in an end product that has a higher SSI and is less elastic than the individual components. Moreover, if different materials are used in a multilayer bandage the elasticity of each layer varies and the net effect becomes very different from individual layer. Adhesive or cohesive layers (which affix to themselves) will also increase the stiffness of a bandage. New bandaging systems are emerging to address the recommendation for an increased SSI compared with traditional short-stretch bandages. For example multilayer compression systems are available where short-stretch bandages are used in combination with adhesive or cohesive bandages. These layering systems aim to increase the rigidity of the LCB and as such, the systems exhibit higher working pressures. Long-stretch bandages are rarely used as a primary treatment modality in lymphoedema but may be used in combination with short-stretch bandages to increase the SSI of an application. One study has examined the use of semi-rigid alginate bandages on weekends as an alternative to short-stretch bandages during a 4 week course of treatment. Short-stretch bandages can soften over a weekend causing reaccumulation of oedema. Semi-rigid alginate bandages were found to resist fluid reaccumulation over a weekend more effectively than short-stretch bandages however alginate bandages have not been investigated as a primary treatment to date [37].

8.12 Tailoring Bandage Pressure to a Limb

The pressure a bandage exerts is determined by three principle factors:

- Tension in the fabric
- The number of layers applied
- The degree of curvature of the limb

The relationship between these three factors is determined by the Law of Laplace. The Law of Laplace states that the pressure applied by a bandage is directly proportional to the tension of the bandage and is inversely proportional to the size of the limb to which it is applied.

$$\text{According to Law of Laplace Pressure}\,\alpha\,\frac{\text{Tension}\left(\text{tension of the bandage}\right)}{\text{Radius}\left(\text{radius of the limb}\right)}$$

Compression bandaging should be applied with a pressure gradient which steadily decreases from the distal to proximal end of the limb to prevent pooling of fluid. Using the Law of Laplace, if bandages are applied at the same tension on a limb where circumference increases from distal to proximal, the pressure will be higher distally and lower proximally creating the desired pressure gradient. The ideal shape of a limb for LCB is a cylindrical shape in cross section and a conical shape along the length of the limb. If a limb is an irregular shape, a graduated compression gradient can be achieved by:

- The use of padding to obtain a more desired shape
- Changing the tension of the bandage
- Varying the number of layers used.

However, in practice, additional pressure may be applied to specific locations. This pressure is achieved by the use of higher density products e.g. stasis pads behind malleoli. Conversely, irregularities such as bony prominences require padding to ensure protection from higher pressures. Padding of irregularities can be achieved with the use of low density products e.g. low density foam. The amount of optimal pressure applied by lymphoedema compression bandaging has not been identified. Research has indicated that in upper limb breast cancer related lymphoedema, lower sub-bandage pressures (20–30 mmHg) appear to be better tolerated than higher sub-bandage pressures (44–58 mmHg) with no significant difference in effectiveness after 24 h wear. The evidence for specific levels of compression required for LCB in people with lower limb lymphoedema is not as strong; however, relatively higher levels of pressure are usually indicated when compared with upper limb LCB. Lower or reduced pressures are used in the long term treatment phase, for night bandaging or in people with palliative conditions. All bandages lose stretchability after application, with repeated use and washing. Damstra and Partsch examined the reduction in sub-bandage pressures in people with upper limb lymphoedema and found 41–48 per cent reduction in pressure 2 h after bandage application and 55–63 per cent reduction in pressure 24 h after bandage application. A bandage applied in a figure of eight pattern produces approximately 1.5–2 times the pressure than the same bandage applied in a spiral pattern with a 50 per cent overlap.

8.13 Effects of Compression

Several studies have shown an impressive reduction in swelling as a result of compression [38, 39], but few have tried to elucidate the mechanism of action for this improvement. The following mechanisms may explain how compression reduces volume in a lymphoedematous limb:

- reduction in capillary filtration
- shift of fluid into non-compressed parts of the body
- increase in lymphatic reabsorption and stimulation of lymphatic transport
- improvement in the venous pump in patients with veno-lymphatic dysfunction
- breakdown of fibrosclerotic tissue.

Reduction in capillary filtration: Starling's hypothesis states that the exchange of water and small molecules is governed mainly by the transcapillary hydrostatic and colloid osmotic pressures. External compression increases the interstitial pressure and prevents fluid from filtering out of the capillary network [40–42]. The role of capillary reabsorption is still a matter of debate. Compression removes more water than protein from the tissue, increasing oncotic tissue pressure and reinforcing the need for sustained compression [43]. In chronic lymphoedema, therefore, success depends on continued compression.

Shift of fluid into non-compressed parts of the body: Oedematous fluid may be shifted into non-compressed distal and proximal parts of the body. Bandaging the fingers and toes and, as far as possible, using compression devices to cover proximal, non-oedematous areas of an extremity should prevent this. Manual lymphatic drainage is especially important in patients with proximal lymphoedema.

Increase in lymphatic reabsorption and stimulation of lymphatic transport: Decongestive lymphatic therapy reduces microlymphatic hypertension and improves microlymphatic dynamics in patients with lymphoedema of the lower limbs. It has been shown that microlymphatic pressure can be nearly normalised with at least 2 weeks of intensive manual lymphatic drainage and multi-layer short-stretch bandaging [44]. In this study a reduction in the maximum dispersion of a fluorescent dye indicated that drainage from the superficial lymph capillaries had improved.

Olszewski cannulated superficial lymph collectors in lymphoedematous and healthy human legs [45]. Using a pressure recorder, flow meter and test tube to collect lymph, the influence of an elastic bandage and contracting calf muscle (exercise) on lymph pressure and flow were measured. The results showed that both compression bandaging and exercise stimulated the movement of stagnating lymph through the lymph collector in lymphoedema patients, in which the lymphatic trunks are filled, but not in healthy individuals, in which they are empty. This supports the conclusion that compression is likely to be more effective when the intrinsic pump fails than when it is functioning normally [7].

Lymphoscintigraphy has been used to demonstrate an immediate increase in lymph drainage after manual lymphatic drainage [46] and the initiation of intermittent pneumatic compression devices [47]. If compression bandaging is continued (using interface pressure 40–60 mmHg), the dynamics of the cutaneous lymphatic circulation remain improved [48]. However, lymphoscintigraphy has shown that several weeks of compression therapy improve disturbed lymph drainage only in some cases and not in patients with severe, indurated lymphoedema [49].

Improvement in the venous pump in patients with veno-lymphatic dysfunction: In cases with accompanying venous insufficiency compression therapy reduces venous reflux and promotes venous return. Inelastic, short-stretch bandages applied with tension to deliver a high pressure can reduce ambulatory venous hypertension [50], resulting in a reduction in capillary hypertension [51] and consequent reduction in the lymphatic load. Subfascial lymph transport is decreased in patients with deep vein thrombosis and postthrombotic syndrome [52], but this can be improved by the application of inelastic bandages [53].

Breakdown of fibrosclerotic tissue: Although the mode of action at the molecular level is not clear, compression also helps to break down fibrosclerosis. In patients with venous leg ulceration compression accelerates blood flow in the microcirculation, favours white cell detachment from the endothelium and prevents further adhesion of the neutrophils. In lipodermosclerotic areas where skin perfusion may be reduced due to the strain associated with high tissue pressure, compression therapy can increase this gradient and improve blood flow. This leads to softened skin.

In a clinical trial the quantitative expression of the genes encoding CD14, interferon-γ receptor (IFNγR), tumour necrosis factor-alpha (TNF-α), very late antigen-4 (VLA-4), TNF receptor-1 (TNFR1) and CD44 was examined in patients with peripheral leg lymphoedema to investigate the potential role of gene expression in the inflammatory response [54]. The findings suggest that proinflammatory cytokines and receptors for growth factors are upregulated in patients with primary and secondary lymphoedema and become downregulated after decongestive lymphatic therapy using a combination of skin care, manual lymphatic drainage, compression therapy and remedial exercises. It seems reasonable to assume that the development of fibrosclerosis in these patients is triggered by the dysregulation of these molecular mechanisms.

8.14 Lymphoedema Compression Bandaging Treatment Programs

8.14.1 Intensive Therapy

During intensive therapy phase a combination of treatments (skin care, MLD, exercise and LCB) is undertaken daily. The frequency of treatment and the degree of compression are adapted for each person depending on the severity of their lymphoedema. The greatest volume reduction is usually seen in the first week of LCB treatment. However, intensive treatment is commonly carried out over a period of 2–4 weeks to allow reductions to continue and then stabilise. LCB is commonly applied to the whole affected limb. If only part of the limb is bandaged, the bandage must extend beyond the area of swelling and may need to include the knee or elbow to prevent movement of fluid into these joints. Pressures greater than 45 mmHg are commonly used to bandage the lower limb.

If there is no limb volume reduction during the first week of intensive therapy, treatment should be re-evaluated to determine the cause of this unexpected result and to modify the treatment program accordingly. Standard intensive therapy can be modified in terms of the level of compression applied and frequency of application.

- Level of compression—Conditions commonly requiring reduced bandage pressure include mild arterial disease, neurological deficits, lipoedema, palliative conditions or lymphoedema in those who are frail or elderly. The oedema reduction achieved with modified intensive therapy may be slower. Standard intensive therapy can be modified to reduce the bandage pressure so treatment is better tolerated.
- Frequency of application—Concurrent medical, mobility or transport issues may limit people from attending daily treatment sessions. Treatments may then be

reduced to less frequent sessions such as second daily. Cohesive or adhesive bandages may be required to prevent the bandage from slipping between visits. More frequent visits may be required during the first week of treatment when the oedema loss is greatest.

8.14.2 Transition Phase

The transition phase aims to consolidate the effects of the intensive treatment phase, to maintain oedema reduction, and to ease the person into the long term management phase. During this phase a combination of LCB and compression garments may be required to reduce fluctuations and prevent swelling from recurring i.e. rebound swelling. A transition phase may also be instituted to balance resource needs with volume reduction maintenance whilst awaiting delivery of a compression garment. During the transition phase the use of therapy-led treatments should gradually decrease and the use of self-management strategies should gradually increase. Treatments used in this phase may include LCB and/or compression garment, skin care, self lymphatic drainage, exercise, MLD and IPC.

8.14.3 Long Term Management

In the long term management phase the focus of control is moved from the clinician to the person with lymphoedema. Compression garments are the primary compression modality used in the long term management phase. Ongoing LCB may be required in the longer term with people who have:

- swelling reduction not maintained by other treatments
- fragile or ulcerated skin
- difficulty tolerating or applying compression garments
- swelling in end of life palliative conditions.

Service availability may limit the capacity for long term bandaging. If ongoing bandaging is required, self or carer bandaging can be taught where appropriate.

8.15 Types of Compression

Compression therapy systems aim to provide graduated compression to the limb or area, acting on the venous and lymphatic systems to improve venous and lymph return, and reduce oedema. Historically, long or short-stretch bandaging, multilayer lymphoedema bandaging (MLLB) and compression garments were the main types of compression therapy used. However, two-layer lymphoedema bandaging and short-stretch strapping systems (Velcro strapping systems—VSS) have been introduced more recently.

Appropriate bandage selection and effective application are important to maintain the patient's normal function and mobility, and to improve concordance with treatment regimens. Patients should be able to walk in comfort with bandaging in place so that muscle contractions in the leg can assist in the movement of lymph.

8.15.1 Long-Stretch Bandages

Long-stretch or elastic bandages contain elastic fibres that enable stretching, in some cases up to 30 cm and more [32]. These bandages have the greatest capacity to stretch in a horizontal manner, with only minimal stretch vertically to allow for some movement of the limb. Because of the bandage's ability to stretch, it does not achieve the same stiffness or rigidity as short-stretch bandages when applied in multiple layers. Long-stretch bandages stretch as oedema increases and provide little resistance to calf muscle contractions. Long-stretch bandages and layered bandages, in particular, provide continuous pressure, with little variation between resting and working pressures.

The use of long-stretch bandages is becoming less popular in the management of lymphoedema since the range of compression achievable can result in inconsistency between practitioners. However, there are indications for the use of such bandages, including to achieve a slower reduction in limb volume in the presence of other comorbidities. For example, in the presence of cardiac insufficiency, increasing fluid volume in the circulation could result in cardiac failure. Other instances when a slower reduction in limb volume may be indicated include where the patient is immobile or has a fixed ankle joint and their calf muscles are not able to act as a pump and/or they have venous insufficiency [55]. Long-stretch bandages are generally used in multiple layers.

8.15.2 Short-Stretch Bandages

Short-stretch or inelastic bandages are recommended to treat a limb that is at least 20% larger than the unaffected limb or that has lost its shape. Short-stretch bandages extend horizontally and retain some elastic component. The ability of these bandages to stretch up to 5 cm allows for movement [32]. Short-stretch bandages produce a stiffer or more rigid encasement of the limb compared to long-stretch bandages. This increased stiffness or rigidity produces a higher working pressure, encouraging venous return and lymph absorption [36].

In contrast to long-stretch bandages, short-stretch bandages produce a lower resting pressure and are less likely to constrict the limb on relaxation [56]. This means the bandages are comfortable for the patient to wear because of their tolerable resting pressures; however, it should be noted that many patients who have chronic oedema and whose tissues have hardened find all compression treatment comfortable because it starts to soften these hardened tissues; this is more comfortable for the patient and encourages better mobility and drainage. It is the stiffness or rigidity achieved by applying layers of bandages in a single application rather than the elasticity of the bandages that is of interest [56].

8.15.3 *Multilayer Bandaging Systems*

Multilayer bandaging systems (MLLB) is recommended to treat a limb that is at least 20% larger than the unaffected limb or has lost its shape. MLLB is a fundamental component of compression therapy for the treatment of lymphoedema. It is used as part of an intensive treatment strategy aimed at reducing limb size, softening hardened fibrotic tissues and correcting any shape distortion caused by disproportionate swelling [57].

8.16 Contraindications to and Instances Where Caution Is Recommended for Multilayer Lymphoedema Bandaging

Contraindications:

- Cellulitis.
- Circulatory problems such as severe arterial disease.
- Ankle-brachial pressure index (ABPI) less than 0.8 and greater than 1.2.
- Unstable cardiac failure.
- Acute deep vein thrombosis.

Caution is recommended when the following apply:

- Existing medical conditions, for example diabetes, rheumatoid arthritis or mild heart failure.
- Motor or sensory deficit.
- Known skin allergies or sensitivities.

MLLB generally involves the use of short-stretch or inelastic bandages. The usual skin care regimen should be carried out before compression is applied. Positioning of the patient or limb during application of compression bandaging is important to ensure mobility. The bandages should not restrict movement or cause the patient discomfort [36]. Technique is important when applying compression from the dorsum of the foot up the leg, since without some form of compression on the toe, swelling could be pushed downwards into the toes. Therefore it is essential to apply compression to the patient's toes to prevent swelling or reduce swelling already present. A cotton stockinette is used to provide a protective, absorbent layer between the skin and the other bandages. It should be applied with the coloured line straight since this ensures any fragile skin is not pulled by an uneven weave. A padding layer is used to protect bony prominences, normalise shape and equalise the distribution of pressure.

Short-stretch bandages should be applied with considerable tension to achieve an interface pressure of up to 60 mmHg on the leg [56]. Upper limits of compression in MLLB are determined by a thorough assessment of the patient, patient needs and treatment goals. However, high compression may be counterproductive in that it also compresses lymphatics. The International Lymphoedema Framework suggested MLLB has upper limits of 30 mmHg for the upper limb and 40–60 mmHg for the lower limb. In practice, the compression soon drops as a result of a reduction in oedema of the limb to approximately 30–40 mmHg within 2 h following application of the bandage [56]. To compensate for the reduction in compression, the bandages should be reapplied to keep the levels of compression in an effective range often on a daily basis [57]. This treatment usually takes up to three weeks [36] but, in practice, may take longer depending on the outcome measure and the necessity of waiting for the arrival of bespoke compression garments.

MLLB should only be undertaken following appropriate training [58]. However, patients who do not have complex needs or do not require specialist intervention could be treated as part of a healthcare professional's general role, were training in the use and application of compression bandaging part of statutory training programmes. While compression bandaging has traditionally been considered specialist practice, general nurses have transferable skills and with training are in a prime position to care for patients with lymphoedema. This would increase the availability of lymphoedema specialist nurses to care for patients with more complex needs.

8.16.1 Two-Layer Bandaging Systems

In the treatment of lymphoedema, two-layer bandaging systems are often used to help maintain patient mobility since these bandages are lighter than other bandages, which may be more restrictive. Evidence suggests that the two-layer bandaging system is effective in the treatment of lymphoedema and provides an alternative to MLLB [59]. Two-layer bandaging systems have advantages over MLLB, including reduced slippage and enabling increased joint flexibility. The two-layer bandaging system is designed to achieve the same treatment outcomes as MLLB, but is considerably less bulky, enabling increased patient mobility.

8.16.2 Compression Garments

Compression garments are an integral component of lymphoedema management in every stage of treatment from risk minimisation to long term management. Achieving well fitting, effective garments to manage lymphoedema is imperative, yet at times challenging. In spite of its widespread popularity evidence is still somewhat subjective regarding its effectiveness [60, 61], particularly in relation to arm and upper body oedema.. The style, fabric, size and compression class is determined by the patient's presenting diagnosis and symptoms [61]. Compression garments function by creating external pressure therefore increasing interstitial pressure in the limb. The effects of this pressure are to encourage movement of fluid from compressed areas into uncompressed areas, improve lymph reabsorption through stimulating lymphatic contractions, break down fibrotic tissue in combination with movement and enhance the action of the venous muscle pump.

Compression garments are generally used in maintenance therapy after intensive treatment or following diagnosis of mild (Stage I) to moderate (Stage I–II) limb lymphoedema [31]. Maintaining the improvement achieved during intensive therapy is challenging. Rebound oedema is common and requires effective compression solutions. The oncotic pressure of the interstitium is increased because compression reduces the water filtration more than the protein content of the tissue. As a result, sustained compression should be continued for maintenance. Compression garments are usually worn daily, from morning to late evening, to benefit from any muscle activity resulting from normal movement and exercise. Muscle activity that occurs against a semi-rigid structure, in this case a compression garment, and the pressure peaks produced from limb movement or the pulsation of arteries also influence the contraction of lymphangions, aiding lymphatic drainage [62].

Compression garments and indications for use

Compression class	Indications for use
Class 1 (light)	Mild varicosis. Varicosis in pregnancy. Mild or early lymphoedema. Lipoedema. Prophylaxis. Maintenance therapy. Palliative care.
Class 2 (medium)	Moderate to severe lymphoedema. Pronounced varicosis. Post-traumatic swelling. After healed minor leg ulceration. After thrombophlebitis. More severe varicosis in pregnancy. Stabilisation after sclerotherapy
Class 3 (strong)	Severe lymphoedema. Post-thrombotic venous insufficiency. Dermatosclerosis. After healed severe leg ulceration. Recurrent leg ulceration once healed.
Class 4 (very strong)	Chronic severe lymphoedema Elephantiasis.

Compression garments are often worn 24 h a day for a period of up to 6 weeks following any bandaging or intensive treatment [32]. Compression garments are measured in terms of mmHg. There is a British Standard available for leg garments only, as well as European standards, referring to both French and German standards. The class of compression garment selected is determined by the patient's condition as well as by comorbidities and contraindications. Healthcare professionals have a role in ensuring that compression garments fit correctly and are comfortable and encourage long-term use to improve quality of life for patients with lymphoedema.

Contraindications to the use of compression Garments [32]

- Arterial disease, depending on severity.
- Congestive heart failure.
- Septic phlebitis.
- Weeping dermatitis.
- Advanced peripheral neuropathy.

Aside from the class or strength of compression garments, there are two main methods of construction: flat and round knit.

8.16.3 Flat Knit

Flat knit garments are constructed by knitting side to side and are then sewn together to form the garment. The size and contours required are achieved by the number of stitches. This type of garment is usually made of a robust fabric and is used in more complex and severe cases (Stages II to III) of lymphoedema [31]. The stiffness or robustness of the fabric means that these garments are less likely to 'slip' into skin folds causing a tourniquet effect, which would increase pressure and lead to tissue damage. For this reason, flat knit garments are often used to help correct shape distortion or following intensive treatment with MLLB so that the patient's limb is supported in a more rigid garment to encourage the skin to regain elasticity and tone [56].

8.16.4 Round Knit

Round knit garments are usually softer in nature and considered less robust than flat knit garments. They are constructed on a set of needles in a circular, continuous knit, and the size of the garment is achieved by altering the number of stitches [57]. This limits what can be achieved in terms of shaping and hence the inability to be made to 'contour' around any shape distortion. This type of garment is usually avoided when there are skin folds and is rarely used if the patient presents with shape distortion. Patients often prefer round knit garments since they are more aesthetically pleasing.

8.16.5 Short-Stretch Strapping Systems

Short-stretch strapping systems are usually an intensive phase treatment alternative to bandaging, but can also be used by patients following training, as a method to maintain their oedema. Often termed VSSs by nature of the use of velcro straps, short-stretch strapping systems are increasingly being used as an alternative to MLLB [63]. Systems such as CircAid, Juxta-Fit, FarrowWrap and ReadyWrap can be used instead of and sometimes as well as bandaging. These systems may be used with a compression garment as an alternative to bandaging to provide opportunities for patients to self-manage a periodic intensive regimen of treatment [63].

A VSS provides high working and low resting pressures, applying approximately 30–40 mmHg depending on the type and structure of the fabric used [63–65]. The systems can be altered as the oedema reduces and reapplied after dressing changes. They are washable and, in accordance with infection control principles, can be reused.

The use of VSSs requires less dexterity to apply than compression garments or bandaging. Patients can learn how to use these systems, and relatives or carers can be involved in care. For patients with large skin folds and misshapen limbs, MLLB remains the first option for treatment, but depending on the patient's circumstances and their ability to take part in their treatment, they might be able to apply VSS while using particular techniques and equipment to ensure compression is still effective [63].

Wound exudate can be managed effectively using VSSs, with most highly absorbent dressings able to lock in exudate and remain in place under the VSS [63]. The VSS can be removed so that the dressing may be changed as required, improving the management of exudate.

Worn over compression garments, for instance on the foot, a VSS can increase the stiffness and therefore rigidity of the garments. This increases compression to areas where the tissues have undergone secondary changes, which have resulted in the lymphoedema becoming more difficult to manage with a single compression garment [63].

This treatment strategy is complex and should only be used by lymphoedema specialists when there are no contraindications for the patient. VSSs offer the opportunity for lymphoedema specialists to use compression in new and innovative ways to treat patients with lymphoedema and in doing so promote independent living while still providing access to professional care. Contraindications to the use of VSS and cases where caution is warranted.

Contraindications to short-stretch strapping

- Infection and acute inflammatory episode.
- Severe peripheral arteriosclerotic disease.
- Decompensated heart failure.
- Deep vein thrombosis.

Caution is recommended with the following:

- Peripheral neuropathy.
- Diabetes.

8.17 Lymphoedema in India

Data regarding the exact distribution of secondary lymphoedema cannot be quoted with certainty but Filariasis can be clearly said as the leading cause followed by breast cancer related lymphoedema. India bears one third of the world's lymphatic filariasis disease burden. Lymphatic Filariasis (LF) is a mosquito-borne communicable disease, classified as a neglected disease of the poor by the WHO because there is little support for research and treatment [66]. The Global Alliance for the Elimination of LF (GAELF) has plans to achieve its goal of the elimination of LF by 2020 [66, 67]. However, these morbidity reduction plans are still in their infancy and there is no public health treatment programme. However, in India, the Institute of Applied Dermatology (IAD) developed an integrative treatment combining the benefits of western biomedicine and the traditional Indian practice of Ayurveda and yoga to treat large numbers of lymphoedema patients in Indian villages. Compression bandaging is part of IAD's integrative treatment of lymphoedema.

There are a wide range of compression bandages which are available in India as an over the counter product though there use sometimes is indistinguishable from those used for venous disorders. The main available product is the long stretch bandage and the cost varies from 10 to 80 USD. In India, physiotherapists are the compression professionals, but they are scarce, even in cities. Biomedical doctors do not go to rural areas, which led the Government to create special courses in rural medicine. However, as each primary health centre (PHC) in India has a minimum of one nurse, primarily because they are paid better, they, along with Ayurvedic paramedical workers, are trained in compression therapy. Unfortunately, areas remain where lymphoedema patients have no access to professional expertise; consequently, the IAD has implemented a compression program to endemic villages, which relies heavily on the training of family members to provide compression [68]. This training comprises sessions on figure of eight bandaging, how to prevent constriction caused by rolling back of bandages, and careful use of moulds for extra pressure as advocated by Foldi [69] and Moffat [70]. At each follow up, patients are asked to demonstrate self compression to identify and where necessary, rectify deficiencies in care giver's skill.

Short-stretch bandaging in combination with long stretch bandaging has a definite role in reshaping distortions, particularly when lymph is drained and the protuberances begin to hang. These are held firmly in place using short stretch, as long stretch bandages in such situations either cause excoriation or constrict their stalk. However, short stretch bandages alone do not stay on top of the distortions and slip into the crevasses causing constriction, and long stretch bandages induce a ballooning effect and occasionally worsen distortion. Therefore, to manage different presentations of lymphoedema in India health care providers have used long stretch and short stretch bandages in combination. Whenever donated bandages are not available, sponge moulds are filled to stabilise distorted oedematous protuberances. Although economical, sponge and moulds frequently cause excoriation and induce bacterial entry points. Continued compression over these superficial abrasions will run the risk of precipitating non healing wounds.

Wearing bandages has social stigma in India; in particular, parents of unmarried girls find it difficult to get alliances in the arranged marriage system prevalent in rural areas. Bandages are not acceptable in fishing or farming communities during work hours. In our tropical climate, sweat and heat generated by long hours of compression, often forces patients to remove the bandages.

Feedback from the community units and the Kasaragod centre of IAD (where patients from 18 Indian states attend) shows usage pattern of compression bandaging. Estimated hours of daytime wear ranges from 0 h (manual workers) to 10 h (housewife, blue collar worker), and at night, range was from 1 h (pensioner), to 10 h. Repeated patient education sessions and telephone counselling are necessary to improve the self care compression delivery, otherwise it is not uncommon to see patients coming back with constriction and wearing the same bandages during cellulitis and worsening lymphoedema. The products available on the Indian market do not meet all the needs of lymphoedema patients, and they are expensive, hence patients and care givers have to be content with the available quality and products. Unfortunately, they do not meet the needs of tropical climate, so innovations are needed, for example, washable bandages with inner absorbable padding. Compression therapy products available on Indian market are too expensive for patients to buy. Long stretch bandages are sold on a par with the short stretch selling price in Europe and America. Patients continue to use long stretch bandages even after elasticity is lost.

Thus in Indian scenario compression therapy has special challenges due to tropical climate and resource-poor settings not fully met by available products in the market.

Best Practice Recommendations for compression therapy in lymphoedema

- Selection of compression therapy should be based on the severity of disease and the individual's preferences and tolerance for therapy. (Grade B)
- Before applying compression therapy the individual's arterial status should be assessed by performing a comprehensive clinical assessment and an ABPI or TBPI. A vascular specialist should be consulted before applying compression therapy to an individual with an ABPI <0.8 and compression is contraindicated if ABPI is <0.5. (Grade A)
- Assessment should include checking for contraindications and conditions in which compression therapy should be used with caution. (Grade A)
- Compression therapy should be applied at a sub-bandage pressure of at least 45 mmHg for individuals with ISL stage II or greater lymphoedema. (Grade A)

8.18 Conclusion

Compression therapy is an essential component of the decongestive lymphatic therapy strategy to manage patients with lymphoedema. The features of lymphoedema and staging of the condition are important considerations when selecting appropriate treatment. Long and short-stretch bandages, MLLB, two-layer lymphoedema bandaging, compression garments and short-stretch strapping systems are commonly used in the treatment of lymphoedema. Healthcare professionals require knowledge of the properties of each system as well as their indications and contraindications, application and associated nursing care to ensure optimum patient outcomes and improved quality of life.

Other treatment options used in conjunction with compression therapy or as individual components include skin care, exercise, manual lymphatic drainage, pneumatic sequential pump therapy and therapies involving laser treatment and deep oscillation. While compression bandaging has traditionally been considered specialist practice, general nurses have transferable skills and with training can care for patients with lymphoedema.

References

1. Handley WS. Two cases of lymphangioplasty for the brawny arm of breast cancer. Proc R Soc Med. 1908;1.(Clin Sect:186–90.
2. Rockson SG. The unique biology of lymphatic edema. Lymphat Res Biol. 2009;7(2):97–100.
3. Brorson H, Ohlin K, Olsson G, Nilsson M. Adipose tissue dominates chronic arm lymphoedema following breast cancer: an analysis using volume rendered CT images. Lymphat Res Biol. 2006;4(4):199–210.
4. Brorson H, Ohlin K, Olsson G, Karlsson MK. Breast cancer-related chronic arm lymphoedema is associated with excess adipose and muscle tissue. Lymphat Res Biol. 2009;7(1):3–10.
5. Warren AG, Brorson H, Borud LJ, Slavin SA. Lymphoedema: a comprehensive review. Ann Plast Surg. 2007;59(4):464–72.
6. Levick JR, Michel CC. Microvascular fluid exchange and the revised Starling principle. Cardiovasc Res. 2010;87(2):198–210.
7. Mortimer PS, Levick JR. Chronic peripheral oedema: the critical role of the lymphatic system. Clin Med. 2004;4(5):448–53.
8. Planas-Paz L, Lammert E. Mechanical forces in lymphatic vascular development and disease. Cell Mol Life Sci. 2013;70(22):4341–54.
9. Breslin JW. Mechanical forces and lymphatic transport. Microvasc Res. 2014;96:46–54.
10. Browse NL, Stewart G. Lymphoedema: pathophysiology and classification. J Cardiovasc Surg. 1985;26(2):91–106.
11. Larsen OA, Lassen NA, Quaade F. Blood flow through human adipose tissue determined with radioactive xenon. Acta Physiol Scand. 1966;66(3):337–45.
12. Smahel J. Adipose tissue in plastic surgery. Ann Plast Surg. 1986;16(5):444–53.
13. Ryan TJ. Lymphatics and adipose tissue. Clin Dermatol. 1995;13(5):493–8.
14. Casley-Smith JR, Gaffney RM. Excess plasma proteins as a cause of chronic inflammation and lymphodema: quantitative electron microscopy. J Pathol. 1981;133(3):243–72.
15. Gaffney RM, Casley-Smith JR. Excess plasma proteins as a cause of chronic inflammation and lymphoedema: biochemical estimations. J Pathol. 1981;133(3):229–42.
16. Zampell JC, Aschen S, Weitman ES, Yan A, Elhadad S, De Brot M, et al. Regulation of adipogenesis by lymphatic fluid stasis: part I. Adipogenesis, fibrosis, and inflammation. Plast Reconstr Surg. 2012;129(4):825–34.
17. Aschen S, Zampell JC, Elhadad S, Weitman E, De Brot M, Mehrara BJ. Regulation of adipogenesis by lymphatic fluid stasis: part II. Expression of adipose differentiation genes. Plast Reconstr Surg. 2012;129(4):838–47.

18. Levi B, Glotzbach JP, Sorkin M, Hyun J, Januszyk M, Wan DC, et al. Molecularanalysis and differentiation capacity of adipose-derived stem cells from lymphoedema tissue. Plast Reconstr Surg. 2013;132(3):580–9.
19. Greene AK. Epidemiology and morbidity of lymphoedema. In: Greene A, Slavin S, Brorson H, editors. Lymphoedema. Cham: Springer; 2015. p. 33–44.
20. DiSipio T, Rye S, Newman B, Hayes S. Incidence of unilateral arm lymphoedema after breast cancer: a systematic review and meta-analysis. Lancet Oncol. 2013;14(6):500–15.
21. Armer JM, Stewart BR. A comparison of four diagnostic criteria for lymphoedema in a post-breast cancer population. Lymphat Res Biol. 2005;3(4):208–17.
22. Brorson H, Hoijer P. Standardised measurements used to order compression garments can be used to calculate arm volumes to evaluate lymphoedema treatment. J Plast Surg Hand Surg. 2012;46(6):410–5.
23. Tassenoy A, De Strijcker D, Adriaenssens N, Lievens P. The use of noninvasive imaging techniques in the assessment of secondary lymphoedema tissue changes as part of staging lymphoedema. Lymphat Res Biol. 2016;14(3):127–33.
24. Cornish BH, Ward LC, Thomas BJ, Bunce IH. Quantification of lymphoedema using multifrequency bioimpedance. Appl Radiat Isot. 1998;49(5–6):651–2.
25. Burnier P, Niddam J, Bosc R, Hersant B, Meningaud JP. Indocyanine green applications in plastic surgery: a review of the literature. J Plast Reconstr Aesthet Surg. 2017;70(6):814–27.
26. Andrade M. Clinical diagnosis: general overview. In: Lee B, Bergan J, Rockson S, editors. Lymphoedema. Cham: Springer; 2011. p. 83–8.
27. Bull RH, Gane JN, Evans JE, Joseph AE, Mortimer PS. Abnormal lymph drainage in patients with chronic venous leg ulcers. J Am Acad Dermatol. 1993;28(4):585–90.
28. Guex JJ. Physiopathology of post-thrombotic syndrome. Update 1994. J Mal Vasc. 1994;19(1):12–6.
29. Peled AW, Slavin SA, Brorson H. Long-term outcome after surgical treatment of lipedema. Ann Plast Surg. 2012;68(3):303–7.
30. Maclellan RA, Zurakowski D, Grant FD, Greene AK. Massive localized lymphoedema: a case-control study. J Am Coll Surg. 2017;224(2):212–6.
31. International Society of Lymphology. The diagnosis and treatment of peripheral lymphoedema. Consensus document of the International Society of Lymphology. Lymphology. 2003;36(2):84–91.
32. Macmillan Lymphoedema Academy. Teaching material. 2014. www.macmillanlymphoedemaacademy.org.uk.
33. Partsch H, Moffatt C. An overview of the science behind compression bandaging for lymphoedema and chronic oedema. In: International Lymphoedema Framework (2012) Compression therapy: a position document on compression bandaging. Best practice for the Management of Lymphoedema. 2nd ed. Saint-Étienne: Imprimerie Reboul; 2012. p. 12–23.
34. Haid H, Lofferer O, Mostbeck A, Partsch H. Lymph kinetics in the postthrombotic syndrome under compression bandages. [German]. Med Klin. 1968;63(19):754–7.
35. Bräutigam P, Földi E, Schaiper I, Krause T, Vanscheidt W, Moser E. Analysis of lymphatic drainage in various forms of leg edema using two compartment lymphoscintigraphy. Lymphology. 1998;31(2):43–55.
36. International Lymphoedema Framework. Compression therapy: a position document on compression bandaging. Best practice for the management of lymphoedema. 2nd ed. Saint-Étienne: Imprimerie Reboul; 2012. www.lympho.org/mod_turbolead/upload//file/Resources/Compression%20bandaging%20 -%20final.pdf. Accessed 23 Dec 2015
37. Kasseroller RG, Brenner E. A prospective randomised study of alginate-drenched low stretch bandages as an alternative to conventional lymphologic compression bandaging. Support Care Cancer. 2010;18(3):343–50.
38. Sitzia J, Sobrido L. Measurement of health-related quality of life of patients receiving conservative treatment for limb lymphoedema using the Nottingham Health Profile. Qual Life Res. 1997;6(5):373–84.

39. Badger CM, Peacock JL, Mortimer PS. A randomized, controlled, parallel-group clinical trial comparing multilayer bandaging followed by hosiery versus hosiery alone in the treatment of patients with lymphoedema of the limb. Cancer. 2000;88(12):2832–7.
40. McNeely ML, Magee DJ, Lees AW, et al. The addition of manual lymph drainage to compression therapy for breast cancer related lymphoedema: a randomized controlled trial. Breast Cancer Res Treat. 2004;86(2):95–106.
41. Johansson K, Albertsson M, Ingvar C, Ekdahl C. Effects of compression bandaging with or without manual lymph drainage treatment in patients with postoperative arm lymphoedema. Lymphology. 1999;32(3):103–10.
42. Badger CM. A study of the efficacy of multi-layer bandaging and elastic hosiery in the treatment of lymphoedema and their effects on the swollen limb, PhD Thesis. London: Institute of Cancer Research; 1997.
43. Partsch H, Clark M, Bassez S, et al. Measurement of lower leg compression in vivo: recommendations for the performance of measurements of interface pressure and stiffness: a consensus statement. Dermatol Surg. 2006;32(2):224–32.
44. Melhuish JM, Clark M, Williams R, Harding KG. The physics of sub-bandage pressure measurement. J Wound Care. 2000;9(7):308–10.
45. Partsch H. Understanding the pathophysiological effects of compression. In: EWMA position document. Understanding compression therapy. London: MEP Ltd; 2003. p. 2–5.
46. Moffatt C, Morgan P, Doherty D. The lymphoedema framework: a consensus on lymphoedema bandaging. In: EWMA focus document: Lymphoedema bandaging in practice. London: MEP Ltd; 2005. p. 5–9.
47. Földi M, Földi E, Kubik S, editors. Textbook of lymphology for physicians and lymphoedema therapists. San Francisco, CA: Urban & Fischer; 2003.
48. Marston W, Vowden K. Compression therapy: a guide to safe practice. In: EWMA position document. Understanding compression therapy. London: MEP Ltd; 2003. p. 11–7.
49. Macdonald JM, Sims N, Mayrovitz HN. Lymphoedema, lipedema, and the open wound: the role of compression therapy. Surg Clin North Am. 2003;83(3):639–58.
50. Thomas S, Nelson A. Types of compression bandage. J Wound Care. 1998;7(8 Suppl):5–10.
51. Clark M. Compression bandages: principles and definitions. In: EWMA position document. Understanding compression therapy. London: MEP Ltd; 2003. p. 5–7.
52. Leduc O, Leduc A, Bourgeois P, Belgrado JP. The physical treatment of upper limb edema. Cancer. 1998;83(12 Suppl American):2835–9.
53. Larsen AM, Futtrup I. Watch the pressure – it drops! EWMA J. 2004;4(2):8–12.
54. Földi E, Jünger M, Partsch H. Science of lymphoedema bandaging. In: EWMA focus document. Lymphoedema bandaging in practice. London: MEP Ltd; 2005. p. 2–4.
55. Quéré I, Sneddon M. Adapting compression bandaging for different patient groups. In: International Lymphoedema framework compression therapy: a position document on compression bandaging. Best practice for the management of lymphoedema. 2nd ed. Saint-Étienne: Imprimerie Reboul; 2012. p. 32–48.
56. Partsch H. Assessing the effectiveness of multilayer inelastic bandaging. J Lymphoedema. 2007;2(2):55–61.
57. Hopkins A. Compression therapy for lymphoedema. Pract Nurs. 2008;19(10):496–503.
58. Macmillan Lymphoedema Academy. Teaching material. 2013. www.macmillanlymphoedema-academy.org.uk.
59. Franks PJ, Moffatt CJ, Murray S, Reddick M, Tilley A, Schreiber A. Evaluation of the performance of a new compression system in patients with lymphoedema. Int Wound J. 2013;10(2):203–9.
60. Johansson K. Evidence for the use of upper body compression garments in patients with lymphoedema. In: Template for practice: compression hosiery in upper body lymphoedema. Aberdeen: HealthComm UK Ltd; 2009. p. 16–20.
61. Lymphoedema Framework. Best practice for the management of lymphoedema: international consensus. London: Medical Education Partnership; 2006.

62. Partsch H, Jünger M. Evidence for the use of compression hosiery in Lymphoedema. In: Lymphoedema framework. Template for practice: compression hosiery in lymphoedema. London: Medical Education Partnership Ltd.; 2006. p. 5–9.
63. Hobday A, Wigg J. FarrowWrap: innovative and creative patient treatment for lymphoedema. Br J Community Nurs. 2013;18(10 Suppl 6):S24.
64. Humen Davey S, Mayrovitz HN. Measuring sub-bandage static and dynamic compression pressures. Symposium, Advanced Wound Care and Medical Forum, San Antonio, April 30–May 3, 2006. 2006. http://clinsoft.org/drmayrovitz/POSTERS-HNM/Poster_SAWC_Pressures.pdf. Accessed 11 Feb 2016.
65. Linnitt N. Compression hosiery versus bandaging for chronic oedema. Nursing & Residential Care. 2011;13(4):183–5. https://doi.org/10.12968/nrec.2011.13.4.183.
66. WHO. The Global Programme to Eliminate Lymphatic Filariasis. 1997. www.who.int/lymphatic_filariasis/disease/en/.
67. World health Assembly. Elimination of lymphatic filariasis as a public health problem. Resolution WHA 50.29. 1997. www.paho.org/English/AD/DPC/CD/psit-lf-wha50-29-eng.pdf.
68. Narahari SR, Ryan TJ, Mahadevan PE, et al. Integrated management of filarial lymphedema for rural communities. Lymphology. 2007;40:3–13.
69. Foldi M, Foldi E, Kubic S. Textbook of lymphology. Munich: Elsevier; 2007.
70. Moffatt C. Compression therapy in practice. Trowbridge: Wounds UK; 2007.

Chapter 9
Compression Therapy Using Low Cost Materials for Managing Different Grades of Lymphoedema in India

S. R. Narahari and K. S. Prasanna

Abstract Lymphoedema and especially secondary lymphoedema resulting from lymphatic filariasis are endemic in India. Extraordinary limb swelling, chronic wounds and pain are among the sequel of this condition. Treatment of this condition is dependent on a good diagnosis and, appropriate compression as developed by a dedicated team of professionals at the Institute of Applied Dermatology in Kasargod, India. This chapter describes the diagnosis and treatment of secondary lymphoedema from filariasis with evidence and assesses the benefits and limitations of its current practice.

Keywords Lymphoedema · Chronic limb swelling · Skin wounds · Lymphatic Filariasis · Integrated medicine

9.1 Introduction

Lymphatic Filariasis manifests primarily as lymphoedema of lower limbs, it is endemic in villages throughout India. Large geographical portions of the country are affected by this disease [1], it is currently claimed by the Government that its effort to eliminate this disease is yielding results. There are many patients with other causes of lymphoedema who are misdiagnosed due to lack of skills and effective tools to identify the aetiology of their condition. Once diagnosed, compression is essential to manage this condition. Providing compression to lymphoedema, a skilled job, and such expertise is not generally available in villages where patients often travel hours to reach a primary health centre. It is heartening to report that since recently, physiotherapy groups are taking interest in Indian cities.

This book is about the importance of compression to manage venous conditions and related complications. The diagnosis and treatment of lymphoedema are central to this aim.

S. R. Narahari (✉) · K. S. Prasanna
Institute of Applied Dermatology, Kasaragod, Kerala, India

R. Mani et al. (eds.), *Compression and Chronic Wound Management*,
https://doi.org/10.1007/978-3-030-01195-6_9

This chapter describes a stepwise clinical approach and practice of compression bandaging in tropical climate and self-care or with family member assistance in a low-income country scenario for different types of presentation and aetiology.

9.1.1 Types of Lymphoedema Requiring Compression

Lymphatic Filariasis is common in India though other such other causes of lymphoedema as congenital lymphoedema, secondary to cancer surgeries; cervical and nodal excision for malignant reasons, post tuberculous adenitis, traumatic lymphoedema, failure of arteriovenous shunt created at cubital region for dialysis, phlebo-lymphoedema, chronic lower extremity wounds, lipoedema, arteriovenous malformations, Klippel Trenaunay Weber syndrome and, breast cancer related lymphoedema have been described and are seen in India. The Institute of Applied Dermatology (IAD) offers a specialist lymphoedema service. In general, the routine treatment of lymphoedema resulting from congestive heart failure, renal dysfunction, hepatic dysfunction (portal hypertension), hypoproteinaemia and hypothyroidism require additional specialized treatment of etiology. Drug induced (e.g. calcium channel blockers, amlodipine, steroids, non-steroidal anti-inflammatories) lymphoedema resolve once offending drugs are withdrawn. Patients with early stages of lymphoedema or immediately after first episode of filarial fever from Kerala are referred to the IAD for diagnosis and, treatment. This is enabled to on account of the high health literacy and better health seeking behaviour of local population. However, there is a large variation in presentations of limb volume and shape in our patients because of huge variations in geographical areas in India [2].

9.1.2 Clinical Assessment Before Bandaging Limbs

1. Lymphoedema staging:

Indian lymphologists follow a seven-stage classification [3]. Our clinic follows international consensus staging for its practical utility for therapists delivering treatments [4]. The International Society of Lymphoedema (ISL) consensus grading followed in clinic is:

Grade I: Pitting oedema may present, this completely resolves on overnight elevation and normal skin.

Grade II (early): Pitting oedema manifests that does not resolve completely on elevation (overnight). Skin is normal.

Grade II (late): Late stages of grade II with non-pitting oedema and thickened skin.

Grade III: Oedema is not pitting with trophic skin changes: Acanthosis, Fat deposits Warty over growth.

2. Limb volume measurements [5]:

Considering limb as a cone and using circumferential measurements taken at different levels is the common method of estimating total limb volume (Fig. 9.1 and Table 9.1). Measurements are also important to anticipate a possible pressure dam-

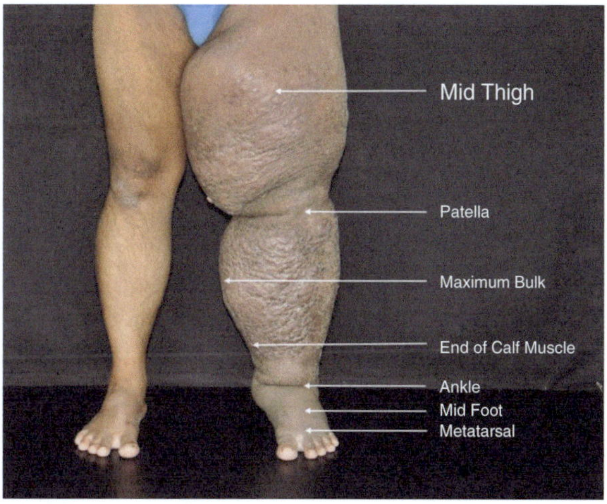

Fig. 9.1 Surface anatomical points on lower limb for circumferential measurements using a tape to estimate the volume of lymphoedema

Table 9.1 Description of limb volume measurement by tape method

Measurement points	Description of measurement
Metatarsal	The circumference of the foot measured in the area that covers the base of the toes
Mid foot	The length of foot is measured from the tip of the great toe to the heel and the middle point is marked. Mid-foot is the circumference at this point
Ankle	The circumference taken around the ankle joint covering both the malleoli, heel and the junction of lower end of the tibia and fibula with the tarsal bones
End-of-calf bulk	The circumference taken at the lower end of the muscle bulk of gastrocnemius
Maximal bulk of gastrocnemius muscle	The middle point of length from the upper end of patella to lateral malleoli
	Is located on the shin. The circumference measured through the maximum bulk of the gastrocnemius muscle in the lying position
Patellar region	The circumference of the affected limb through the popliteal fossa and the middle point of the patella
Mid-thigh	Limb length measured from the anterior superior iliac spine (ASIS) to the upper end of patella. The circumference of the limb through the mid-way is measured
Maximal bulk standing	The middle point of length from the upper end of patella to lateral malleoli
	Gastrocnemius muscle in the standing position using this point

age due to compression therapy. Smaller ankle and calf circumference and exposed bony and tendon areas can quickly develop pressure damages. According to modified Laplace law [6].

3. Water displacement method

The gold standard method for volume measurement is by water displacement method i.e. immersing the lymphoedematous limb in a large bucket up to mid-thigh and the volume of water displaced is measured (Fig. 9.2). As volume of the limb reduces the water displaced by volume measurement decreases as described by the principle of Archimedes which is taught in all high schools. However, the scarcity of water in some geographical areas such as Gulbarga district in Karnataka state makes this method difficult to use. Also, lymphoedema in endemic dry geographical areas are generally limited to knee level [7].

4. Assessment of shape of the limb

Shape distortions of the limb tissue protuberances at different anatomical regions separated over crevasses pose challenges to the therapist during compression. Oedematous tissue over dorsum of the foot over reaching metatarsal region is most difficult to compress. Surface extensor tendons over ankle region is a risk factor for creation of pressure damage. All such features on lymphoedema should be meticulously documented through measurements and photographs to record the response to treatment (Fig. 9.3).

5. Vascular assessment

Compression should never impede or block the arterial circulation to any part of the body and for this reason, a vascular assessment of a patient with lymphoedema is essential. A limb with lymphoedema contains more collagen than it does lymph and this collagen acts as a in-dwelling natural compression stocking underneath the skin in patients with long standing lymphoedema. The arterial vascular status of the legs of all patients with lower limb lymphoedema should be assessed to determine whether compression is indicated and if so, which level. An examination of the dorsalis pedis is the essential first step. Clinically it may be difficult to locate this pulse in lower limb lymphoedema on account of foot swelling—a problem also common in patients with venous leg ulcers. The measurement of ankle brachial pressure index (ABPI) is reliable and, in trained hands, relatively easy to do. ABPI below 0.8 is a contraindication for compression. Compression therapy is recommended to all patients with ABPI greater than 0.8 as discussed in detail in the chapter on surgical solutions in this book.

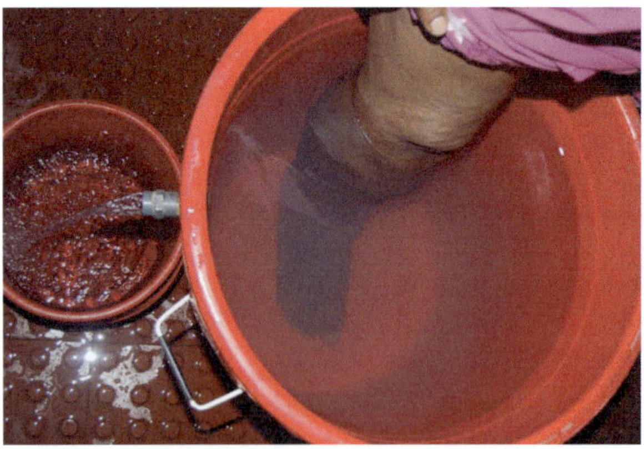

Fig. 9.2 Gold standard method to estimate the limb volume applying Archimedes principle. Displaced water is measured in litres

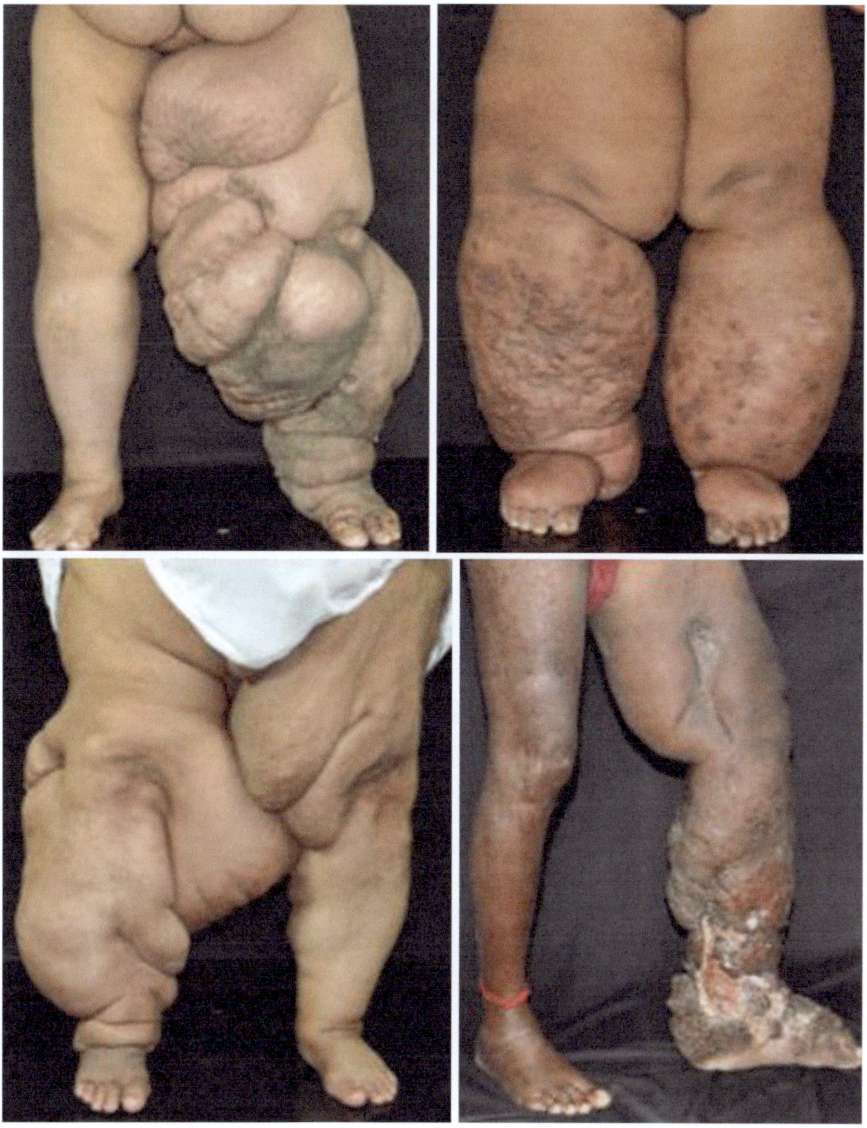

Fig. 9.3 Several patients present with multiple folds and different shapes. Documenting folds and protuberances is important to workout initial compression strategy. Compression methods may have to be changed as treatment progresses and patient's limb size reduces

Briefly, ABPI is measured as follows. The procedure is explained to the patient. To measure the brachial systolic blood pressure place a cuff around the upper arm. Locate the brachial pulse and apply ultrasound contact gel. Holding the Doppler probe at 45 degrees to the skin move the probe to obtain the best ultrasound signal. Inflate the cuff until the signal is abolished then deflate the cuff slowly and record the pressure at which the signal returns and the probe should not move from the site. Repeat the procedure for the other arm. Similarly, ankle pressure is obtained by placing the sphygmomanometer cuff 10 cms proximal to the ankle while recording pressure over the dorsalis pedis artery. Use the highest of the two values to calculate the ABPI.

6. Pain assessment

All patients complaining of chronic limb or wound pain are assessed using specially designed tools of pain measurement. Commonly, the presence of pain in our patients is associated with the presence of non-healing ulcers. All pain scales used to measure severity and improvement due to treatment are used including Wong Baker Faces scale, Visual analogue scale and Numerical rating scale scales. In use these scales are printed on the patient's case sheets. Patients may choose the scale of their choice but should be asked to indicate pain using the same scale during every follow up.

7. Assessment of the skin

It has only recently been identified and emphasised that oedematous skin is unhealthy, in these circumstances, the epidermis itself contributes to the oedema [8]. It is the response of the epidermis to oedema that partially explains lymphoedema and accounts for the benefits of meticulous skin care. In addition to the skin thickness assessment by pinching the skin presence of bacterial entry lesions need to be assessed (Fig. 9.4).

A patient's attendant, may meticulously wash the limbs with soap and water every day for large sized limbs. Self-wash by patients is advocated for those with smaller sized limbs. The wash should include removal of dirt and deposits between skin folds for larger limbs. Following limb wash, the affected limb is immersed in an ayurvedic (an Indian Traditional Medicine system) skin care "*phanta*" solution [9] for 20 min. This solution has an acidic pH. An Ayurvedic doctor selects various herbal powders for preparing "*phanta*": *Manjistha, Sariva, Yestimadhu* and *Triphala,* based on the Ayurvedic principles of treatment. Later the water and moisture contents are dried using a cotton towel with special attention to eliminate moisture from the skin folds. Whenever fungal intertrigo is present, colourless Castellani's paint may be instilled and if it doesn't respond, anti-fungal creams may be tried. Eczematous lesions are treated with topical betamethasone dipropionate 0.05% while wounds, if and when infected, are treated with appropriate antibiotics. Unhealthy granulation tissues and slough on the base of the chronic wound are treated with *Jatyadi thaila* of Ayurveda. Skin care also includes regular cleaning and paring of nails and hair. Patients are strictly advised to use good, well-fitting, cobbler-made footwear [10]. Patients are given an Ayurvedic oil massage using appropriate herbal oils. We have explained the procedures of oil massage and selection of oil in a previous report [7].

8. Assessment of the wound

The aetiology of a chronic lower extremity wound is assessed such as arterial, venous, diabetic, trophic and so on [11]. Ankle mobility, nutritional assessment of

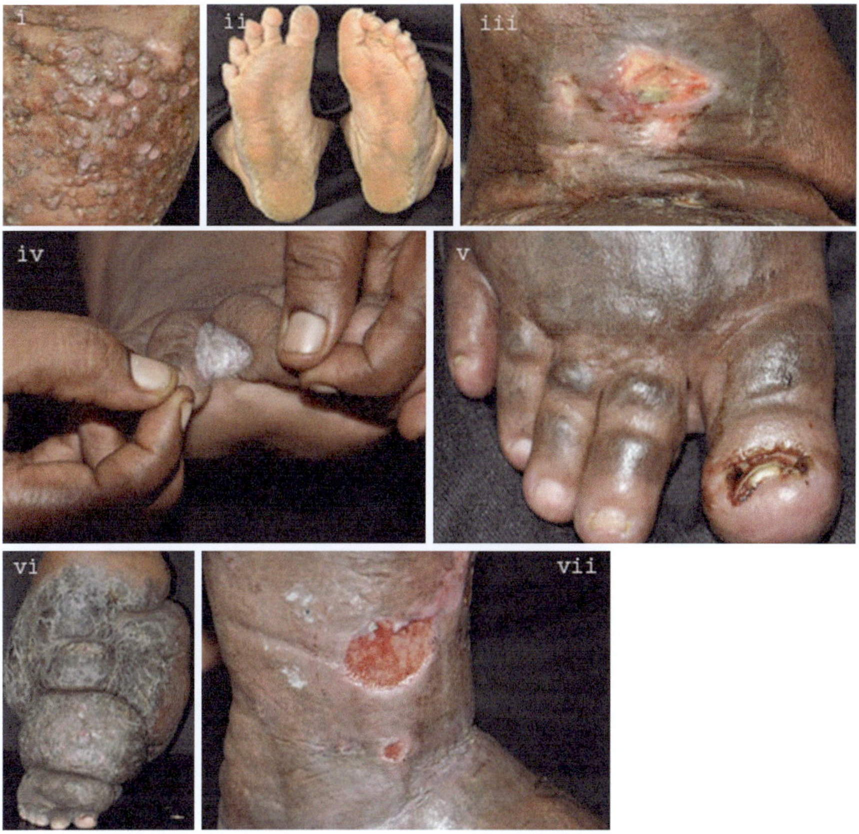

Fig. 9.4 Bacterial entry lesions are the greatest risk for cellulitis (**i**) folliculitis (**ii**) cracked foots (**iii**) excoriation (**iv**) intertrigo (**v**) paronychia (**vi**) eczema (**vii**) ulcer

the body, gait deformity and associated foot disabilities are documented. Signs of inflammation around the wound and actual wound examination are important before compression therapy is initiated. Appropriate wound dressing and care must be given before embarking on compression therapy.

9. Mobility and Range of Motion (ROM) of joints

Patient's mobility and ROM are assessed meticulously. Range of movement is assessed using a goniometer. These are recorded in a video and used during follow up assessments. An example is the 'Lurch' gait observed in lymphoedema patients. This lurch gait results from arresting flexion of the hip and initiating extension; the trunk lurches backward at heel-strike on weakened side to interrupt forward motion of the trunk (Fig. 9.5).

10. Other investigations include blood tests for anaemia, infection, diabetes, general condition such as heart failure or portal hypertension

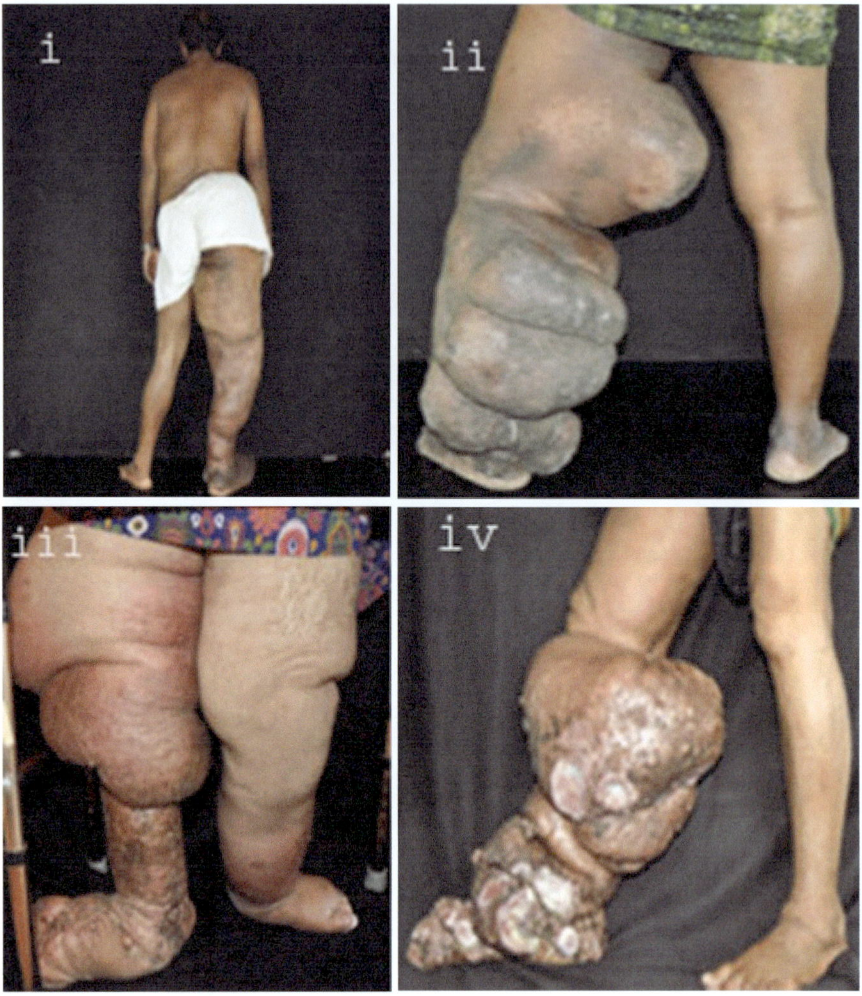

Fig. 9.5 Various disabilities often observed with lymphoedema (**i**) limb length inequality in a patient with arteriovenous malformation with tissue hypertrophy (**ii**) large limb with multiple folds and protuberances (**iii**) outer rotation of hip (**iv**) irregular shape with multiple ulcers limited below knee. Each one of them need customized compression therapy plan

11. Patients should be encouraged to maintain a healthy body weight: Lymphoedema is associated with obesity and obesity is a risk factor for the development of lymphoedema especially after treatment for breast cancer. Although a direct relation is not established in the case of obesity induced lymphoedema, our patients always receive recommendations for diet management

9.1.3 *Low Cost Bandage Materials Available in the Indian Market:* (Fig. 9.6)

1. Finger bandage: Stretching cloth without rubber 6 cm width and 2½ m in length for grade 2 and long stretch elastic rubber knitted bandages 6 cm width and 2½ m in length for grade 3 lymphoedema
2. Cotton cloth
3. Cold cure foam (CCF) sheet
4. Micro cellular rubber (MCR) sheet
5. Chalky bags and moulds
6. Sandwich mould
7. Long stretch bandage: It is available in three sizes 8 cm × 4 m, 15 cm × 4 m and 10 cm × 4 m. The bandage has 1 m of product length stretchable up to 4 m.
8. Short stretch bandage whenever donated from abroad

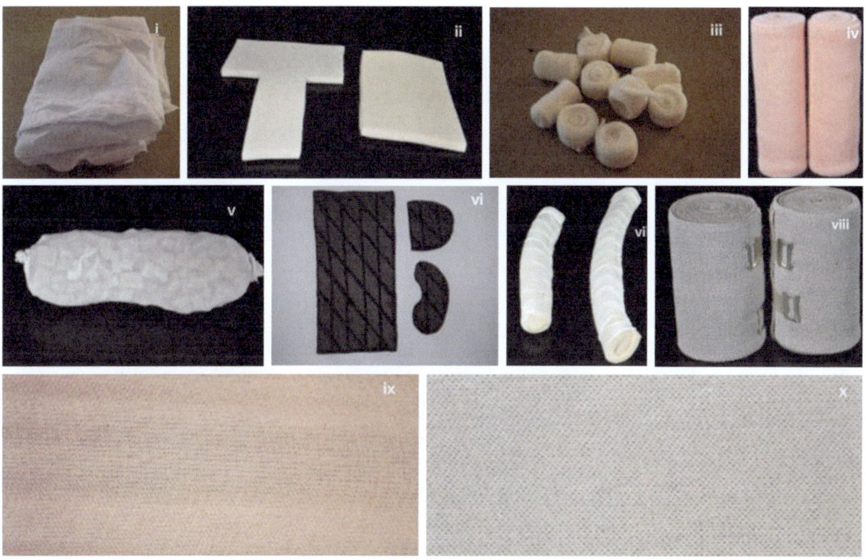

Fig. 9.6 Low cost materials used in preparation of accessories of compression therapy in IAD for low resource set up. (**i**) cotton cloth (**ii**) T shaped CCF sheet (**iii**) finger bandages (**iv**) long stretch cotton bandages (**v**) chalky bag (**vi**) MCR rubber moulds (**vii**) sandwich mould (**viii**) short stretch bandages (**ix**) long stretch fabric while stretching (**x**) fabric while stretching short stretch bandage

9.1.4 Preparation Before Compression

(a) A CCF sheet is cut into long pieces to cover the limb especially in patients with severe deformities as shown in Fig. 9.3. The length and width of material required are determined from the size of the limb (limb girth measurements). Three such pieces are needed for each limb. Three methods used to cover the limb with CCF sheet. *Two pieces in length:* In this method one long piece of CCF is placed on anterior side of the limb and second piece placed over posterior side of the limb. As limb size reduces, we reduce the breadth of the CCF. In *One piece around* method the limb is covered with single piece of CCF. This method is used when the swelling is spherical with multiple deep crevasses and limited below knee. *Two pieces wide* method is used when oedema extends up to groin and there is less oedema in knee region making an hour glass appearance. CCF proportional in measurement to the girth of mid-thigh is covered over thigh region from little above the mid-thigh to knee. Another piece of the CCF is taken as per the measurement of maximum bulk at calf and covered over leg (shin) down till ankle. The pressure should be less in upper segment. These methods are used to avoid constriction at various levels. Current consensus in compression therapy is to limit the used of CCR material to minimum.
(b) Chalky bag: Take remaining of cut sheets of CCF and make into small pieces then fill in to the cotton stockinet and tie it's both ends.
(c) Sandwich mould is prepared using smaller sheets covering them with stretching cloth. Thickness of this type of mould depends on the width of crevasses that are separated using them (Fig. 9.7).

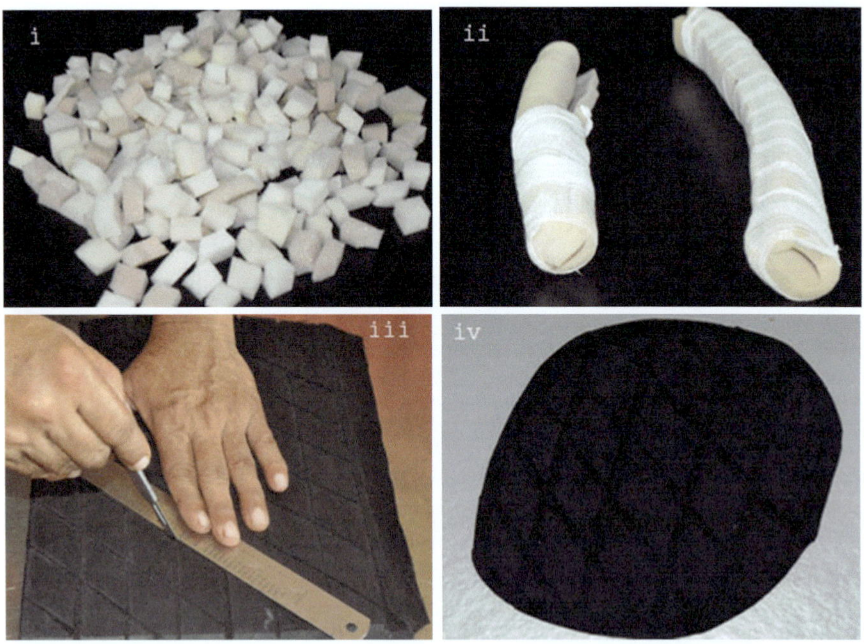

Fig. 9.7 (**i**) CCF pieces for chalky bag (**ii**) sandwich mould on right and partially completed sandwich mould on the left (**iii**) carving diamond shaped grooves on MCR mould to facilitate lymph drainage (**iv**) Microcellular rubber mould

9.1.5 Compression Protocol

Various skilled manual procedure is employed to achieve effective compression.

9.1.5.1 Toe Compression

Oedematous toes are covered with gauze or bandage material after performing the part 2 on Indian Manual Lymph Drainage using Ayurvedic oil [12]. Initially the bandage should be rolled in clockwise to metatarsal region twice then it is rolled over great toe and back over metatarsal region (Fig. 9.8). Later moved to the second toe this bandaging procedure is repeated for four medial toes except the little toe [6]. Toe compression prevents shifting of oedema from foot to toe and acts as a toe separator to reduce intertrigo. Its disadvantage is that it absorbs the moisture thus aggravating intertrigo.

9.1.5.2 Cotton Cloth Wrapping

After toe compression the limb is wrapped by a lining up to the level of oedema [7]. The material should be starch free. Purchased cotton cloth is washed dried, sterilized and used. It is cut and used according to the size needed. Ribbed cotton stockinet is used for those practicing self-compression as it is easier to pull over limb. This is available in different diameters (5 cm, 7.5 cm, 10 cm, 15 cm and 10 m in length). Size is selected according to the thigh measurement. It is easier to use than cotton cloth. It is available in roll and is preferred by patients who can afford the costs. Cotton cloth wrapping prevents the direct contact of oil with compression bandage. The oil that remains on skin following IMLD ruins the elasticity of the compression bandage. The long stretch bandages are made up of elastic fabrics which cause sweat induced occlusion and irritation when in direct contact with skin. Cotton cloth absorbs moisture and sweat reducing folliculitis.

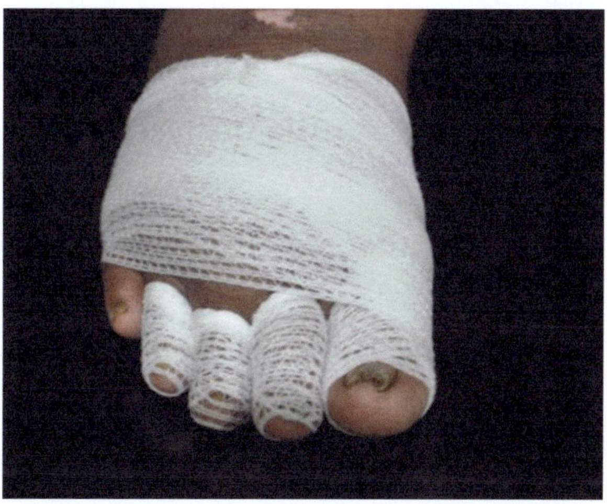

Fig. 9.8 Dorsal view after the toe compression. Little toe is not included in toes compression because it often causes fissures on plantar side at the base of the toe. Toes bandages are applied when oedema is observed over the toes. If toes are free of oedema toe bandages are not applied

9.1.5.3 Sponge Moulds for De-kinking

Without washing off the oil, a patient's limb is covered by cotton cloth. Later folds are filed with suitable mould to get uniform limb shape. Long stretch compression material is wrapped over these moulds in a figure of "8" manner. If the therapist decides to give more pressure over organized regions of limb MCR mould are placed before wrapping with long stretch bandages. MCR moulds are not routinely placed on the first day. Instead they are used on day 3 onwards depending on the need for more pressure. The moulds selected as per the shape of the limb. If the protuberances are large chalky bags or sandwich mould are prepared according the depth of crevasses to separate folds (Fig. 9.9). In certain folds only CCF pieces are inserted.

Mould placing helps free flow of lymph by possibly de-kinking the lymphatic channels. A separated fold is kept dry due to moisture evaporation and reduces the fungal infection. Outer surface of the chalky bag becomes irregular and creates a wavy surface of compressed skin facilitating free lymph flow.

The density of the CCF is 23 and 15 mm its thickness. As Lymphatic filariasis limbs are generally presented in uneven sizes and shape CCF mould of different

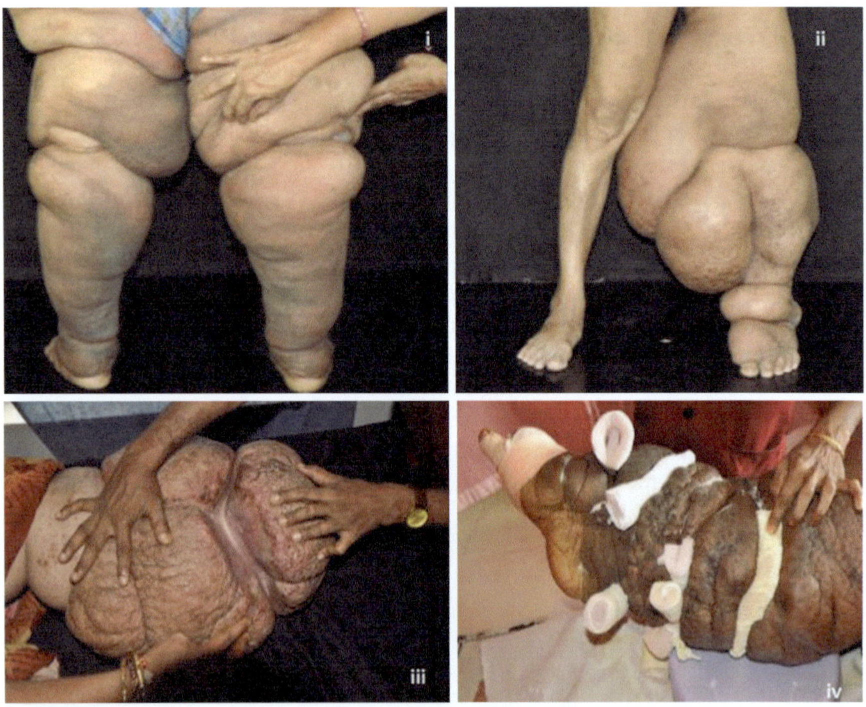

Fig. 9.9 De-kinking lymphoedema folds to facilitate free flow of lymph. (**i**) Lymphoedema folds in a large volume limb (**ii**) Sagging oedema in a patient with multiple folds (**iii**) Deep crevasses with large protuberances of oedema filled tissue (**iv**) placing sponge moulds to keep the folds separated and crevasses open underneath the bandage

sizes and shapes are used. The edges of sponge moulds are cut in slanting manner to avoid excoriation. CCF moulds are generally used over ankle; knee and thigh region. There is more mobility in these areas and maximum chance of constriction. The sponge moulds avoid constriction [5], keeps the limb cylindrical and provides equal pressure as in other areas. A CCF mould is placed in thigh at the upper part of bandage to avoid slipping/rolling of the bandage.

CCF is used to avoid constriction due to rolling back or slipping of bandages into crevasses, to separate the folds to achieve free drainage of lymph and to achieve the uniformity of compression.

9.1.5.4 MCR Moulds for Additional Pressure

Different shapes of moulds such as rectangular, bean and half-moon are used depending on the position and shape of the oedema. Spherical moulds or half-moon shade is used in metatarsal below malleolar region, rectangular shape mould for shin, bean shaped for ankle beneath the malleoli to drain oedema in the region.

9.1.5.5 Preparation of MCR Moulds

A piece of MCR sheet is cut in corrugated manner to create diamond shaped grooves. This gives more pressure and facilitates the lymph flow throw grooves. Initially the MCR of the required shape is taken. Oblige incisions are made using scalpel. The incised lines were broadened so as to create grooves. Edges are blunted to avoid excoriation.

9.1.5.6 Long Stretch Bandages

This bandage is made up of cotton and rubber thread which has 300% extensibility and 100% elastability. Bandages are expensive priced at 5.08US $ and durability is about 2 weeks (Table 9.2). Although products manufactured by over 50 companies are available in the market only Dynamic techno medicals DYNAMIC TECHNO MEDICALS products meet the basic minimum quality of 140% stretch-ability.

9.1.5.7 Short Stretch Bandages

Uniform pressure may be maintained by using short stretch. Compression is done in spiral method as the stretch of the bandage is less and it is difficult to maintain fig of 8. Short stretch compression is done after cotton cloth wrapping. The movement or shifting of oedema to the abdomen is observed frequently while using short

Table 9.2 Disinfection and durability of compression materials

Material (manufacturer)	Durability	Disinfection methods	Cost per unit in INR
Toe bandages—stretch band **(Soft touch)**, Long stretch finger bandage **(Dynamic Techno Medical)**	Reused for 3 days. Long stretch toe bandages can be reused for a month	Washed, ironed or dried, Stretch bandages are disinfected in the same way as long stretch compression bandages	Stretch band: 16 INR (0. 23 US$) Long stretch finger bandage: 50 INR (0.71 US$)
Cotton cloth **(Arual bharth)**	Reused for 2 weeks	Cotton cloth should be washed daily with hot water and dried under sun	INR 25 per meter (0. 3 US$)
Cold cure foam (CCF) sheet **(Spring field)**	Changed every 7 days	Nothing	Per sheet INR. 250 (3.65US$)
Microcellular rubber (MCR) sheet	Reused daily for 1 month or until it gets fully soiled by oil	Nothing	Per sheet INR.510 (7.30US$)
Sponge moulds	Changed every 7th day	Nothing	Depends on the material used
Long stretch bandage **(Dynamic Techno Medical)**	Two weeks as its rubber threads break or lose elasticity when exposed to oil. Otherwise they last for 3 weeks	Washed once in 10 days using cold water & bathing soap. Should not be squeezed or hanged in lane, should be dried under shade by spreading on floor/ paper	INR.355 (5.08US$)
Short stretch	More than long stretch. Patients keep using the same bandage for 3 months	Washing in cold water using bathing soap	Recently introduced to Indian market
Bandage holding hooks	3–4 days for Indian made, European lasts for 1 week	Nothing	Available from local companies on bulk order
Ribbed cotton stockinet-TOP C Net **(Dynamic Techno Medical)** DYNAMIC TECHNO MEDICALS	One piece can be use up to 1 month	Cotton cloth should be washed daily with hot water and dried under sun	5 cm × 10 mt-INR 365(5.22US$) 7.5 cm × 10 mt-INR 490(7US$) 10 cm × 10 mt-INR. 595 (8.52US$) 15 cm × 10 mt-INR895 (12.82US$)

stretch bandages compared to long stretch bandaging in large size limbs indicating quicker lymph drainage. It gives superior results while using over organized limbs. Fixation of bandage is superior to long stretch thus providing constant compression for longer periods. It provides additional pressure and softens the limb.

Short stretch bandages are until recently not routinely available in Indian market.

Compression stockings are available in market in three sizes large, small and medium. We recommend its use after limbs attain normal shape and size.

9.1.6 Position of the Patient for Bandaging

9.1.6.1 Lying Position

To achieve the lying position, the patient should sit on a cot with lower limbs in supine position. This position is used for giving proper compression to foot and shin.

9.1.6.2 Standing Position

In this position patient should stand both limbs apart, one kept one on a small stool of 20 cm height to create space for giving compression over the circumference of the limb (Fig. 9.10).

9.1.6.3 Straight Leg Raising Position

In this method, the patient should lay on cot and supporting staff or patient's family member hold the limb straight up in 90 degrees. This position is used to give compression at mid -thigh particularly for protuberances sagging from thigh region (Fig. 9.11).

9.1.6.4 '*Bhekasana*' Position

Bheka = frog *Asana* = Position (Position like a frog). Patient lies on cot in prone position then the affected leg is bent backwards, compression begins from foot. The position is used for swellings over maximum bulk sagging on to ankle. This method is adopted to open the narrow fold created by the sagging oedema (Fig. 9.12).

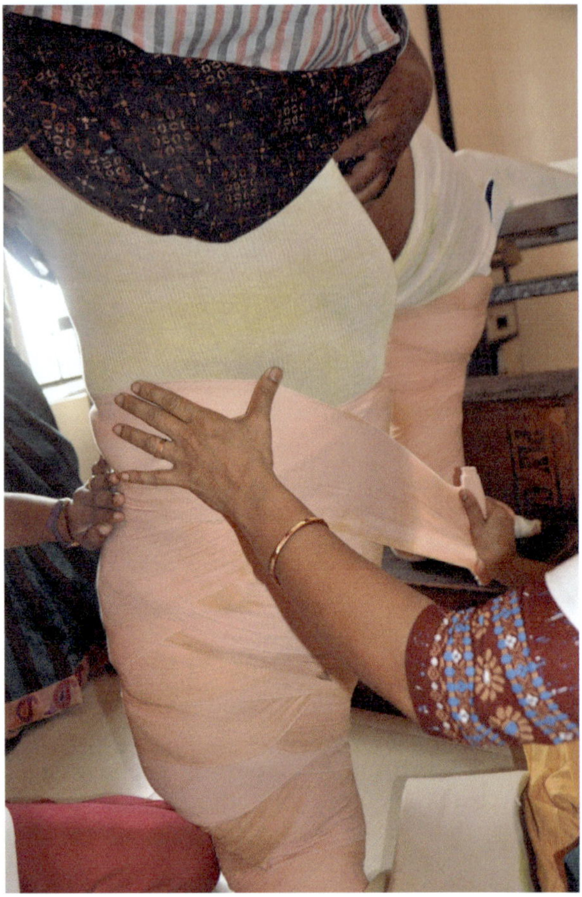

Fig. 9.10 Bandaging lymphoedema in standing position. Note the position of left lower limb kept over the step. This is done to create space for giving compression. Sub-bandage pressure also depends on the stretching of bandage while bandaging the limb

9.1.7 Bandaging Techniques

9.1.7.1 Multilayer Bandaging

First layer of short stretch bandage in spiral manner and over that long stretch bandage in figure of 8. This is used to hold the sagging skin & swelling when oedematous out growth becomes loose following lymph drainage. Whenever large folds give deep crevasses the long stretch slips into such grooves and cause constriction increasing the oedema below such folds (Fig. 9.13).

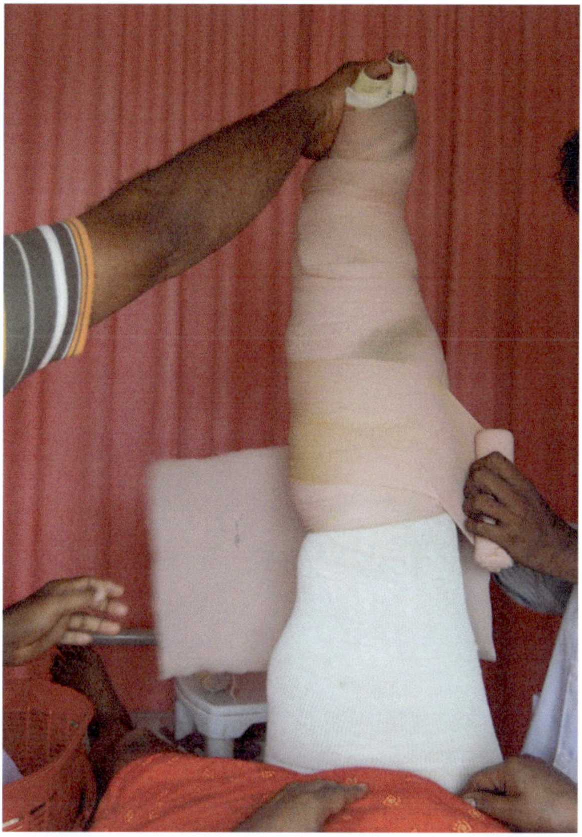

Fig. 9.11 Bandaging lymphoedema in straight leg raising position

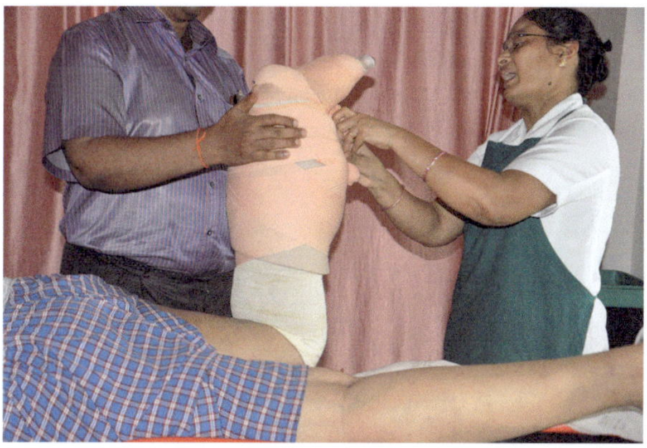

Fig. 9.12 Bandaging lymphoedema using *Bhekasana* position

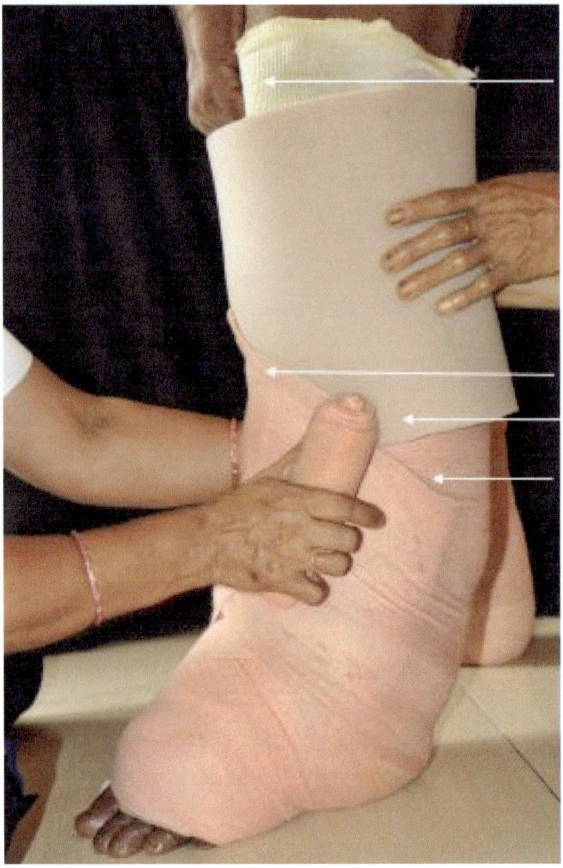

Fig. 9.13 Multilayer bandaging using long stretch bandages and other low-cost accessories. First layer of cotton cloth, second layer by long stretch bandage, a CCF sheet used over an area of likely pressure damage to reduce the sub-bandage pressure, fourth layer is made of long stretch bandage

9.1.7.2 Full Compression

This is a common method of compression given up to groin in figure of 8. It is done when the oedema is up to the groin. In case of unilateral limb, the mid-thigh measurement of both limbs is compared. If affected side of thigh measures more than 10% cm than normal thigh then former is bandaged up to mid-thigh (Fig. 9.14).

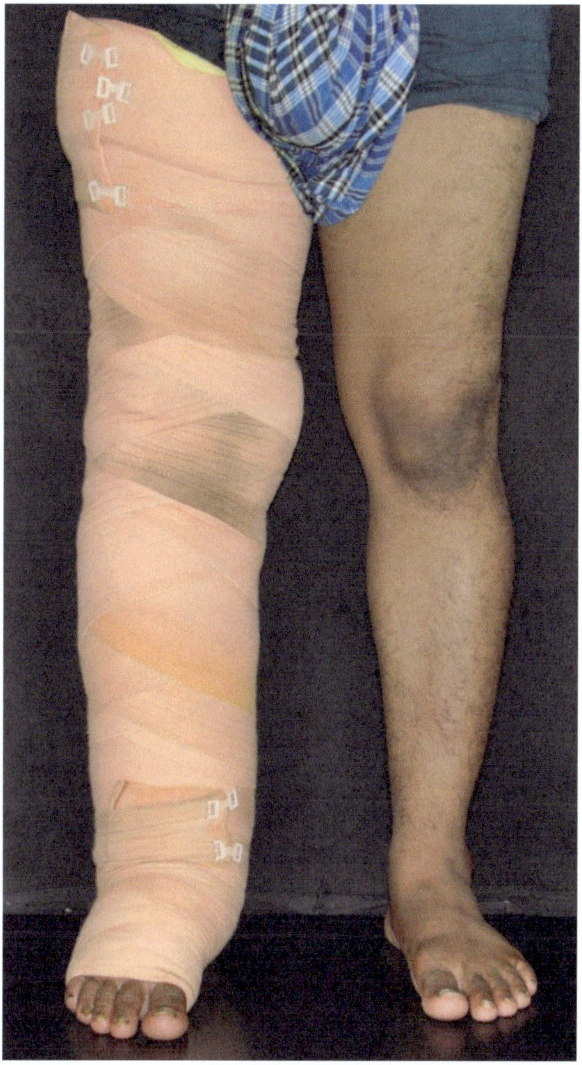

Fig. 9.14 Full compression or thigh length compression. Usually compression bandages are applied till the upper level of lymphoedema. Observe the figure of 8 bandage system, absence of toes compression as patient didn't show oedema over the toes and position of clips used for anchoring bandage

9.1.7.3 Half Compression

In this method bandaging is given only up to knee joint in figure of 8 when the oedema is limited up to knee level. One week after below knee compression, girth measurements are repeated. If the measurement increases in thigh then the compression is extended up to mid-thigh (Fig. 9.15).

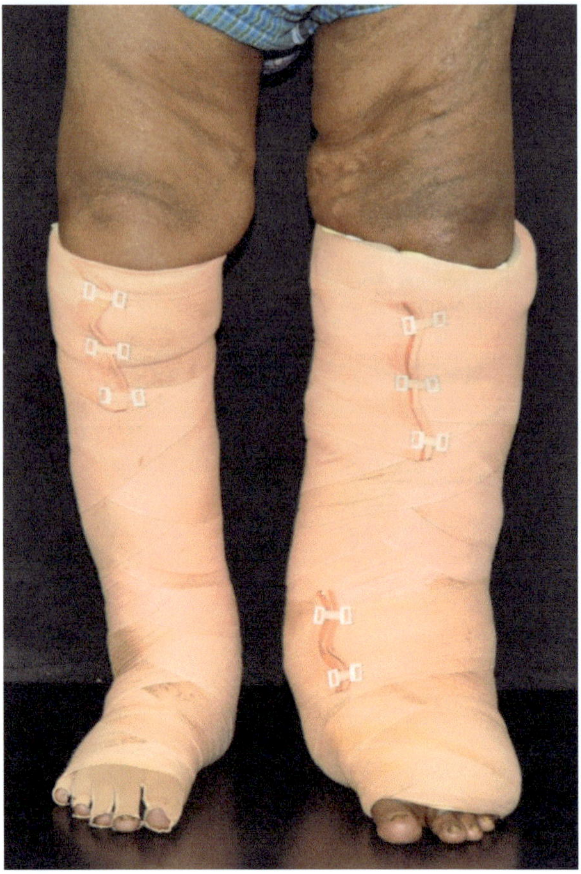

Fig. 9.15 Half compression for lymphoedema limited below knee. Note the presence of toe bandages on the right side and its absence on left side

9.1.7.4 Half & Half compression

Compression is given over the feet and leg and avoiding knee joint; extended till mid-thigh This is practiced when oedema is large over thigh and maximal bulk but minimal oedema over knee joint (Fig. 9.16). Many patients come back with constriction of bandages at popliteal fossa after full compression. Such patients are managed with this compression until the time therapist is able to bring swelling under control. Circumference at patellar region is measured periodically to watch for oedema formation over knee.

9.1.7.5 Forefoot Compression

When oedema is more on foot projecting outwards covering the toes, the bandage is inserted into the crevasses underneath the protruded portion and above the toes and anchored over maleoli, bandage running parallel to sides of heel (Fig. 9.17).

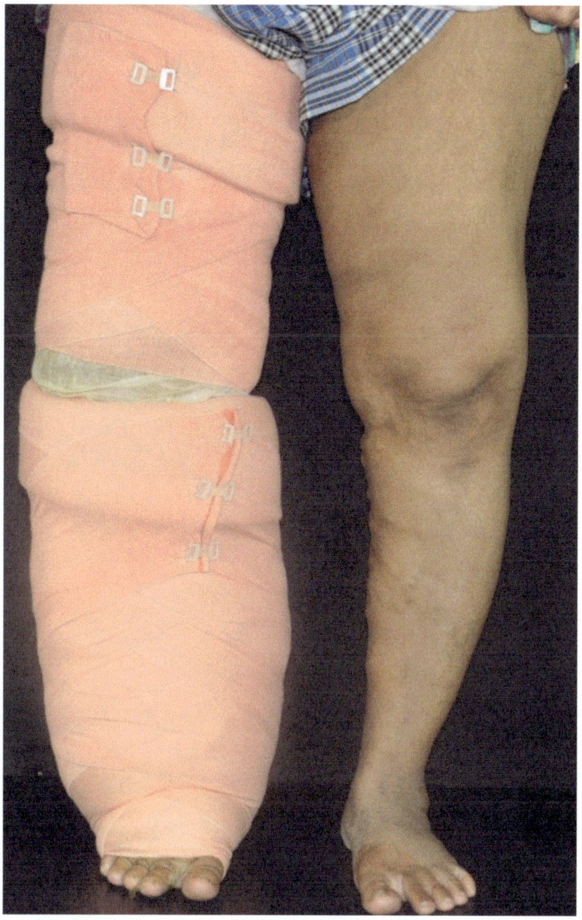

Fig. 9.16 Half and Half compression. This is generally done on irregular shaped limbs with large thigh oedema requiring simultaneous compression on thigh oedema from the first treatment day. Observe varicose veins on the left lower limb. Venous insufficiency is a common occurrence in lymphoedema

9.1.7.6 Ankle Free Compression

Many patients don't get the skill required to make perfect spiral rotation of bandage and anchor it over the ankle. Very often we see pressure damage on anterior portion of the ankle. In such patients' compression that begins at the metatarsal level ends at ankle joint. Then the next bandage begins from malleolar level (Fig. 9.18).

9.1.7.7 Bandaging Over Genitalia

Scrotal oedema doesn't require CCF except when margins of bandages cause excoriation of scrotal skin or at the base of the penis. Long stretch cotton elastic compression material of size 8 × 4 or 10 × 4 cm are used. Scrotal oedema is given compression using technique of scrotal support similar to post-operative bandaging done after hydrocele surgery. Bandage pack generally slips and it is difficult to

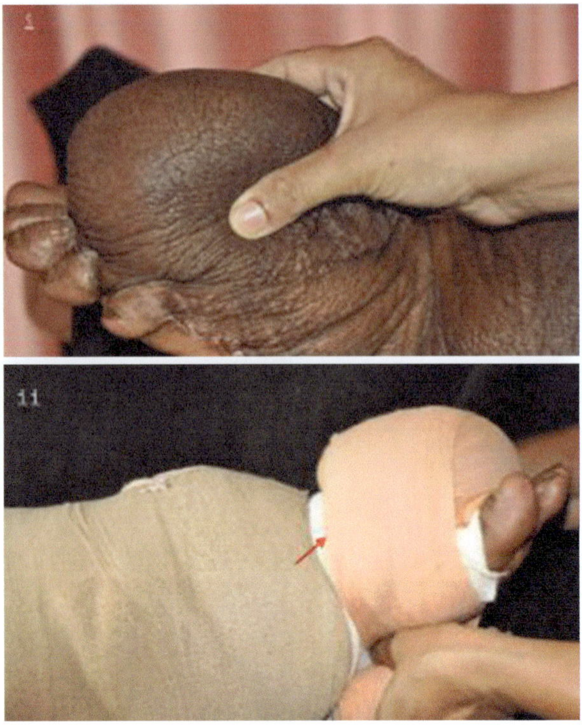

Fig. 9.17 (**i**) Difficult to manage swelling of forefoot requires skilled bandaging. (**ii**) Note the smaller width of the bandage (8 cm) arrow. Note the use of cohesive bandaging system over the leg above ankle. When swelling reduces patients are encouraged to use shoes with lases to give additional compression

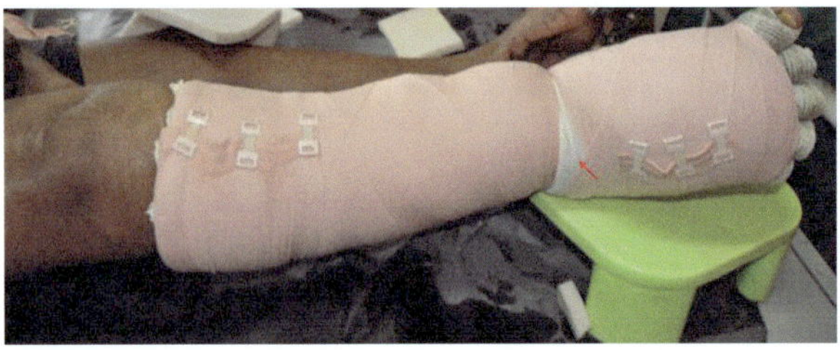

Fig. 9.18 Ankle free bandaging in lymphoedema. In this bandaging technique roll of bandage stops at the base of ankle and next role starts above ankle joint, not a continuous bandaging covering malleoli (arrow). This patient was given below knee bandaging and toe compression

prevent slipping. *Langota* or *Langoti*, a traditional style of Indian loincloth for men, is used above bandaging system to prevent slipping of bandage pack (Fig. 9.19). Patients having genital lymphoedema involving scrotal skin, penis and labia majora require frequent removal of bandages and often changing them because its gets soiled by urine. In such patients we do commonly observe lower abdominal oedema. These are very difficult to drain. Patients are not fully satisfied and they continue to follow up probably because there are limited options to treat.

Compression alone is not sufficient to drain lower abdominal lymphoedema. Our clinical observations have shown that yoga has a role in draining lymph from geni-

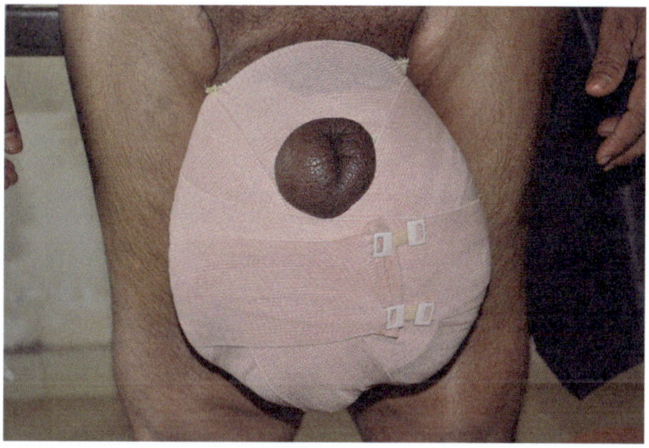

Fig. 9.19 Genital oedema is managed using scrotal support system but using long stretch bandages of 10 cm × 4 m. Repeated counselling is required to improve patient's concordance to treatment. Patients who continue to adhere to treatment regimen improve over the time

talia and lower abdomen [13]. Vaginal compression is given in similar manner as menstrual pads but giving more pressure. We have developed scrotal and vaginal massage systems [14]. Patient's spouse is encouraged to practice the same daily before giving compression.

The bandage material used determines the level of compression achieved and its effectiveness. Short stretch bandages are the preferred bandage for the treatment of primary and secondary lymphoedema. Short stretch bandages cause a higher pressure during activity (working pressure) and relatively low pressure at rest (resting pressure). Padding using cotton and selective use of foam rubber can protect protruding bones and reduce fibrosis. Padding should also protect kinking and closure of lymphatics by compression of deep folds and crevasses.

9.1.8 *Adverse Effects Following Compression Bandaging System*

Especially because of paucity of medical facilities and services in rural India lymphoedema treatment training is often self-care. Although many patient bystanders manage to maintain the compression therapy back home it is common to see pressure damages during follow-up visits alongside reduction in lymphoedema volume. We present a few common examples of pressure damages (Figs. 9.20, 9.21, 9.22, 9.23, 9.24, 9.25, 9.26, 9.27, and 9.28).

9.1.9 *Challenges of Compression Therapy Practice in the Community*

Compression therapy is a complex bandaging system requiring time, patience and skills to learn. Many issues associated with the delivery of compression therapy in Indian rural set up. Assessment of issues affecting concordance to use of

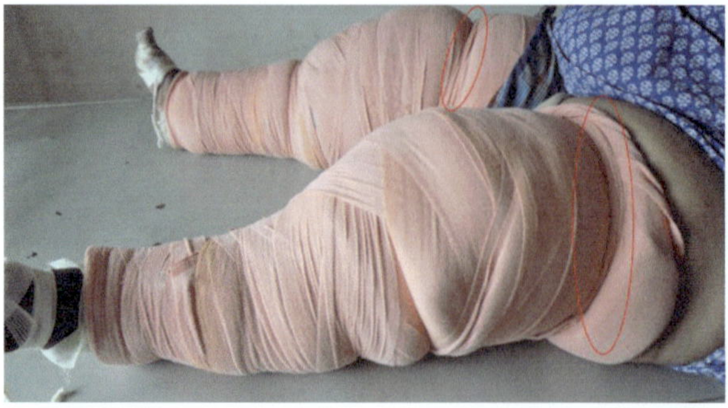

Fig. 9.20 Long stretch bandages often slip into crevasse causing constriction. This is common in patients presenting with large protuberances especially when patients attempt self-care in early stages of treatment. Note patient didn't apply foot compression

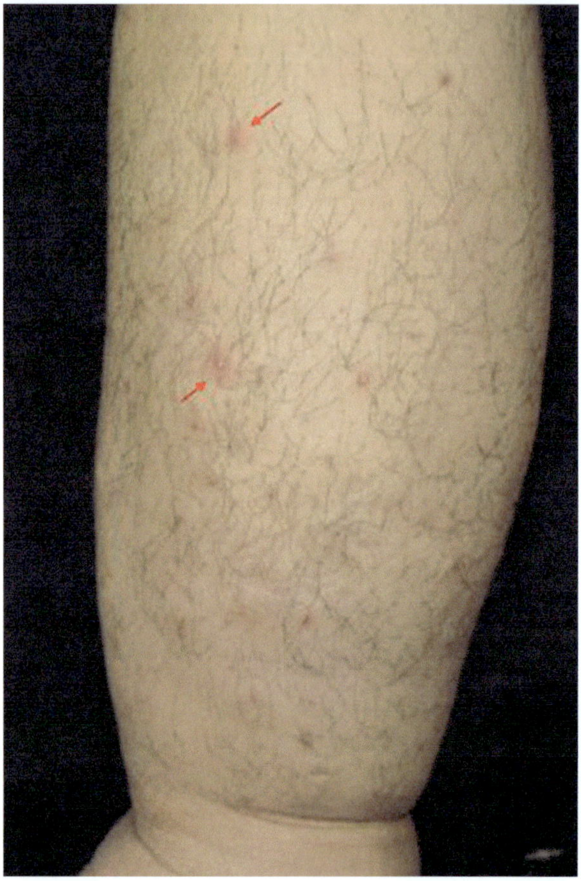

Fig. 9.21 Tropical climate often induces folliculitis (arrow) underneath the bandage pack. This is often aggravated by oil massage

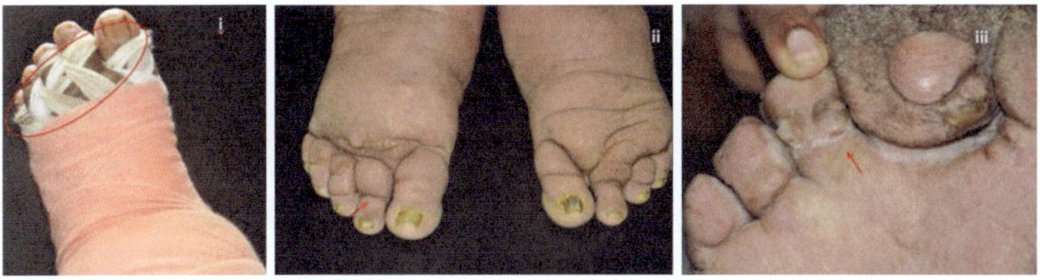

Fig. 9.22 Pressure damage of plantar side of toes occur when (**i**) toes banging rolls back to become a thread at the base of toes. (**ii**) this leads to constriction over the middle of toes (**iii**) also causes a painful fissure giving an additional treatment induced bacterial entry lesion

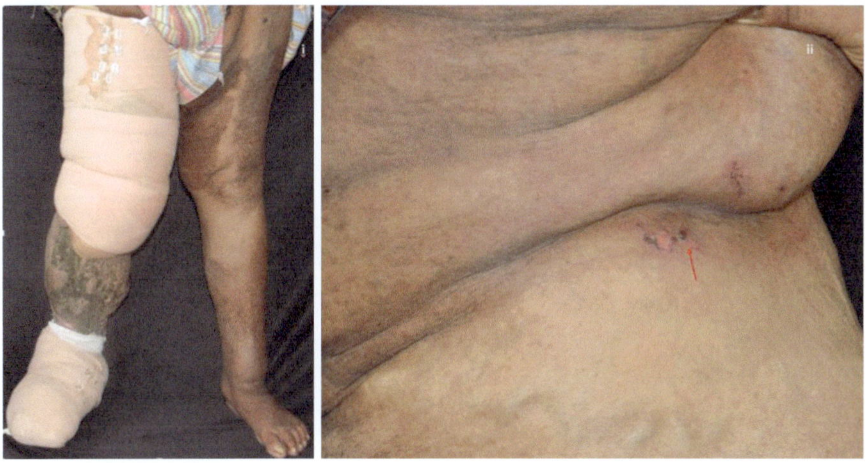

Fig. 9.23 Compression therapy is a challenge in patients with post lymphoedema surgery because of uneven shape and compromised skin on donor and recipient sites (**i**) A patient with post lymphoedema surgery with half and half compression. Compression free area is the site of debulking surgery (**ii**) Friction blisters occur over the edges of creases after walking with bandages (arrow)

Fig. 9.24 Fissure due to dekinking: Protuberances are often firm in consistency and oedema is non-pitting due to desmoplasia. This causes excoriation on the edges of protuberances caused by sponge moulds used to separate crevasse (arrow)

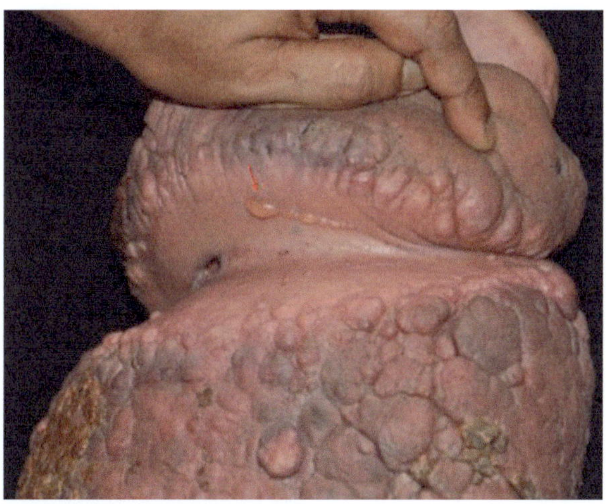

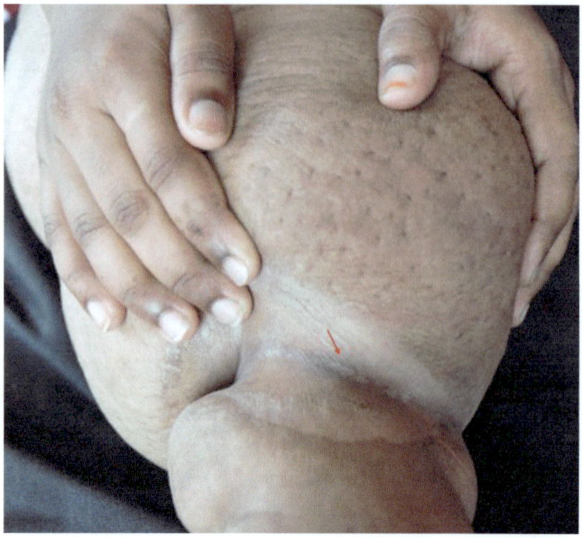

Fig. 9.25 Fissures also happen on the base (arrow) of protuberances due to friction of long stretch bandages while walking

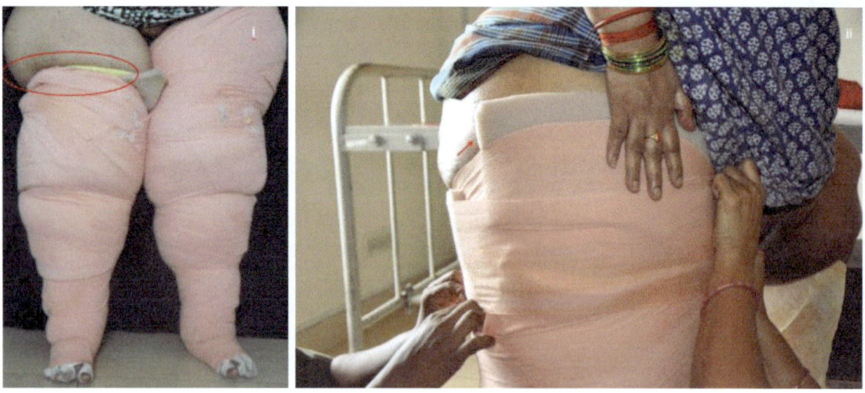

Fig. 9.26 Rolling back of long stretch bandages in upper part cause constriction (**i**). This can be prevented by (**ii**) using a strip of CCF sheet placed underneath the upper end of bandage (arrow)

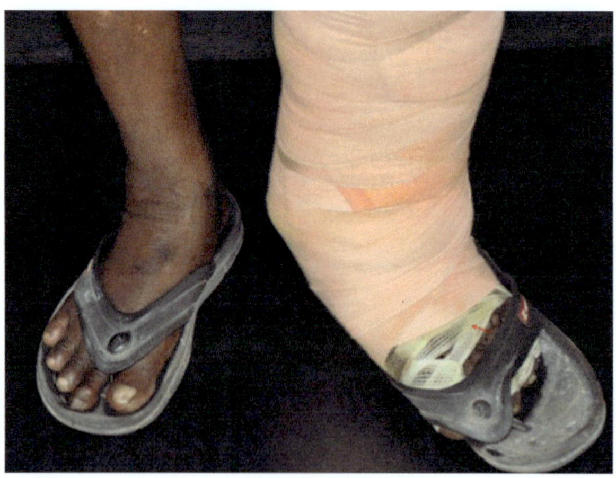

Fig. 9.27 Slippers is a common footwear used by Indians. In lymphoedema patients it is not protective and pushes the bandages backwards (arrow) causing constriction. Due to the non-availability of well-fitting foot wear affected limb's bandage and foot are often unprotected

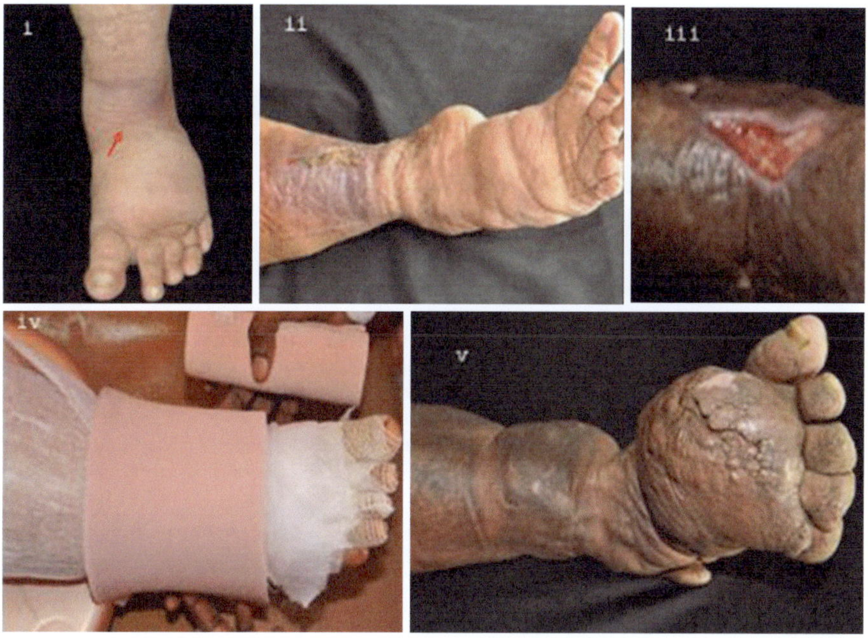

Fig. 9.28 Recognizing early signs of pressure effect is important to prevent pressure damage. Symptom of early pressure damage is burning pain after a few hours of bandaging lymphoedema. Therapists often ignore it after checking blanching at the tip of toes to confirm that circulation is not affected. (**i**) an erythema is noticed over the area immediately after removal of bandage (arrow) and patients' pain is relieved. Next stage would be excoriation (**ii**) followed by ulcer (**iii**). Using CCF moulds over the pressure area under the bandage will reduce sub-bandage pressure and relieves pain (**iv**). In self-care programmes patient manages pain using CCF moulds. If not managed properly over the time a protuberance develops distal to the pressured area (**v**)

compression lifelong is crucial for its success. There is a training need for patients and their family members. Repeated patient education sessions and telephone counselling are necessary to constantly improve the self-care compression delivery (Fig. 9.29). Otherwise it is not uncommon to see patients coming back with constriction and wearing bandages during cellulitis and worsening lymphoedema. This is a challenge in at least 20% of patients who present with large limbs of over 15 L of volume and those with several co-morbidities. They need supervised treatment sessions before such lymphoedema is under control. All kinds of work agrarian, industrial or office jobs begin early morning requiring a person to work through the day. This poses a challenge to devote time early morning for putting on bandage packs and adjusting the same after a short period of walking or routine activity. Often this forces the patients for self-care even while the lymphoedema volume has not reduced sufficiently to qualify for self-care. Sleep disturbance is a common complaint among patients in early stages when bandaging is necessary to be retained overnight. Most lymphoedema patients are resigned to a sedentary life style and dependent on their family before arrival for treatment. Lymphoedema treatment programme requires them to adopt to a new active life style through repeated counselling and motivation.

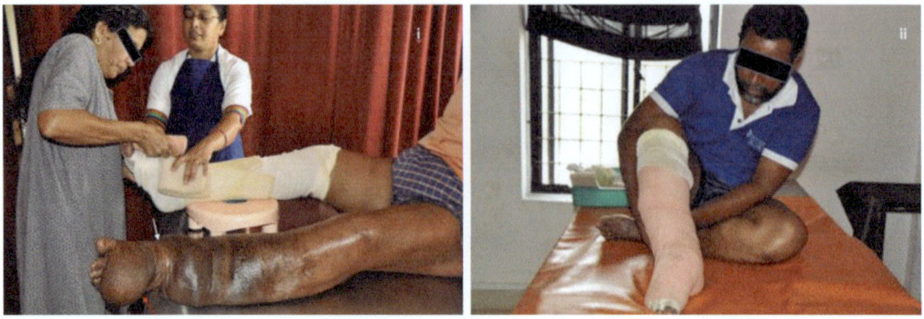

Fig. 9.29 Therapists devote few hours on each patient to educate a family member on compression bandaging (**i**) and patients for self-care (**ii**). Constriction area (white arrow) on left lower limb lymphedema resulting in a newly formed protuberance on the foot (red arrow). Note the presence of Ayurvedic oil over lymphoedema. In integrated treatment compression bandaging is done immediately after oil massage. Oil damages rubber threads and reduces the life of compression bandages

9.1.9.1 Cost of Compression Materials

Bandages and compression garments are very expensive for Indian patients (Fig. 9.30). Inexpensive, durable bandages and garments need to be developed if this important therapy is to become available in resource-poor areas 66–80.7% of material cost of integrated lymphoedema treatment is used for compression therapy. The products available in Indian market are too expensive for patients to buy. Long stretch bandages are sold at par with the short stretch selling price in Europe and America. Patients continue to use long stretch bandages even after its stretch-ability is lost. In our experience products available in Indian market do not meet all the needs of lymphoedema patients.

Some patients don't wear compression during working hours. Especially fishermen, house maid workers, agriculture labourers and construction workers are unable to use the bandage during their work hours (Fig. 9.31). Despite of repeated training several patients are unable to carry out the same and require supervision at home. In a populated country like India this would mean an overstretching service.

9.1.10 Care of Bandages

Bandages get soiled soon especially in rural areas where patients do many different kinds of job including wading through mud and water. Long stretch bandages need cleaning and drying without damaging rubber mesh inside the cotton. Patients were advised to wash the bandages in normal tap water with toilet soap and dry in shades. Bandages should not be hanged up for drying neither dried in sunlight.

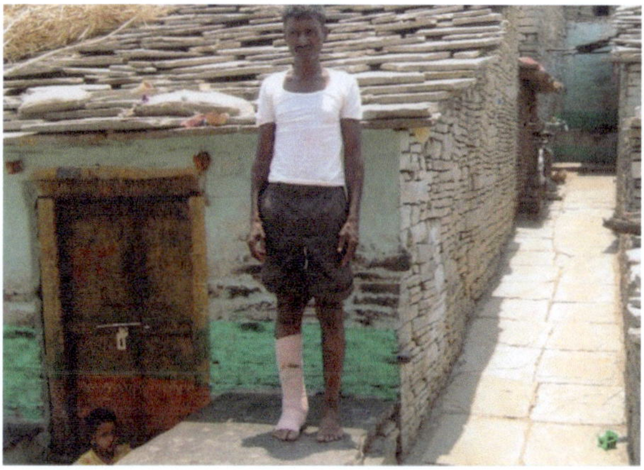

Fig. 9.30 Concordance to compression therapy for lymphoedema was improved during a field trial of integrated medicine for lymphoedema in Gulbarga district of Karnataka through home visits. Lymphatic Filariasis causes lymphoedema and is endemic in Indian villages. Lymphatic Filariasis is the neglected disease of the poor. Note the dwelling condition of this patient in the background

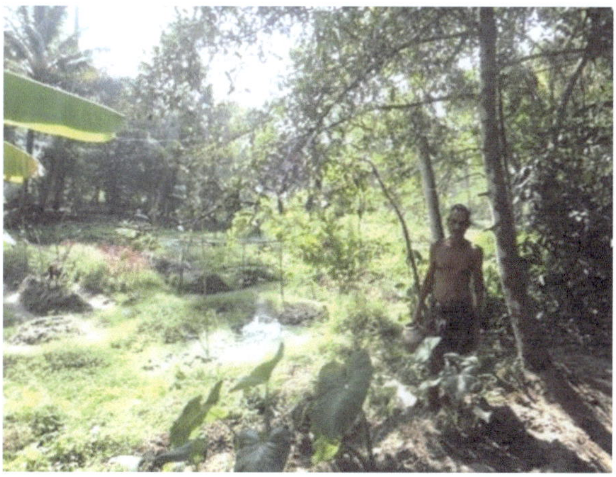

Fig. 9.31 Agrarian workers who are in contact with water and require to fold limbs are not able to use compression therapy during work hours. Lymphatic Filariasis mostly affects such people costing billions of rupees to Indian rural economy

9.1.10.1 Social Stigma and Isolation

Wearing bandages has a social stigma in India, particularly parents of unmarried girls find it difficult to get alliances in the arranged marriage system prevalent in rural areas. Encouraging peer participation in work place improves concordance to treatment (Fig. 9.32). Our efforts to reach compression therapy to the poor and the needy was partially successful. Although many patients re-use the bandages even after complete loss of elasticity their concordance to treatment is fully demonstrated in Fig. 9.33.

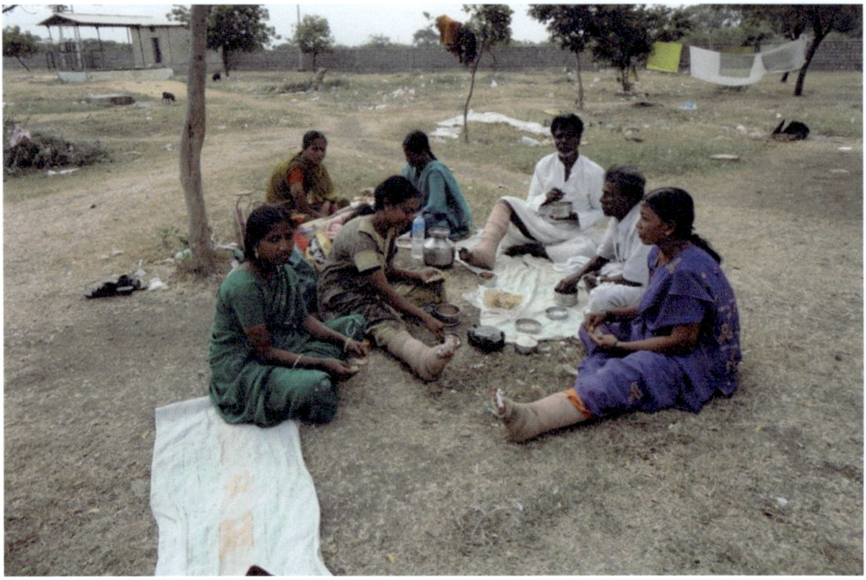

Fig. 9.32 Socialising with bandages for lymphoedema requires motivation and often involving peer patients in their work

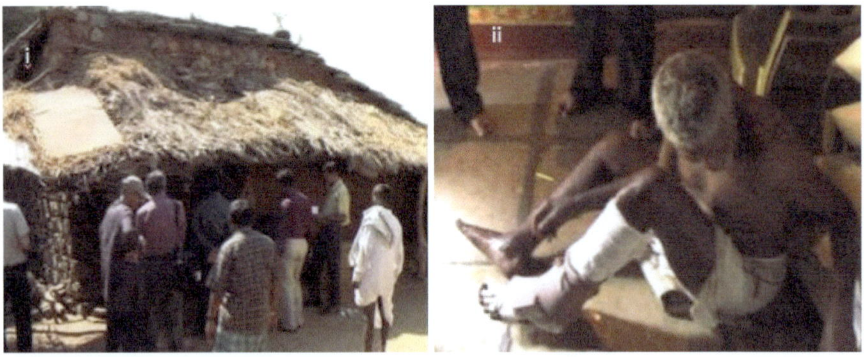

Fig. 9.33 Integrated treatment of lymphoedema was trialled in the villages of Gulbarga district of Karnataka with the support of Government of India. (**i**) Remote village in Sedam Taluk patients living in a hut (**ii**) convinced of its benefits a patient is using worn out compression bandages

The feedback from the community units and the Kasaragod centre of IAD (where patients from 22 Indian states attend) gives the community usage pattern of compression bandaging. Table 9.3 shows estimated hours of retaining compression bandages by patients.

Table 9.3 Compression wearing duration of patients with different socio-economic background as recorded by patients' statement during the follow up at IAD

Occupation		Day time (h)	Night (h)
Fisherman		Not doing	5
Coir worker		Not doing	6
Manual labourer		Not doing	8
Driver		10	6
Office workers		8	9
Unemployed		10	10
Govt. employees		8	10
Housewife		10	8
Farmer/labourers in dry land		5	8
Business	People	10	10
Barbers		10	6

9.1.11 Co-morbidities

Bandaging lymphoedema associated with comorbidities require special attention. Although benefits of compression therapy should be weighed against ability for self-care or family member assisted compression therapy lymphoedema patients with severe co-morbidities are always willing to attempt treatment. Lymphatic Filariasis affects more than one limb and often upper and lower limbs. Compression therapy is extremely embarrassing to patients especially when complete treatment is attempted (Fig. 9.34).

9.1.12 Future Perspective of Compression Therapy for Lymphoedema in India

Research suggested from work done in IAD where appropriate compression therapy is given by trained staff following a good diagnosis includes

- Determination of the correlation between exerted pressure and volume reduction with a view to learning more about the effectiveness of our treatment regime
- Frequency of bandage changes
- How to achieve optimal control of compression delivered when using bandages with slip and this renders retention, difficult.
- Do alternative means of delivering compression described in other chapters in this book offer any value to the patient with lymphoedema

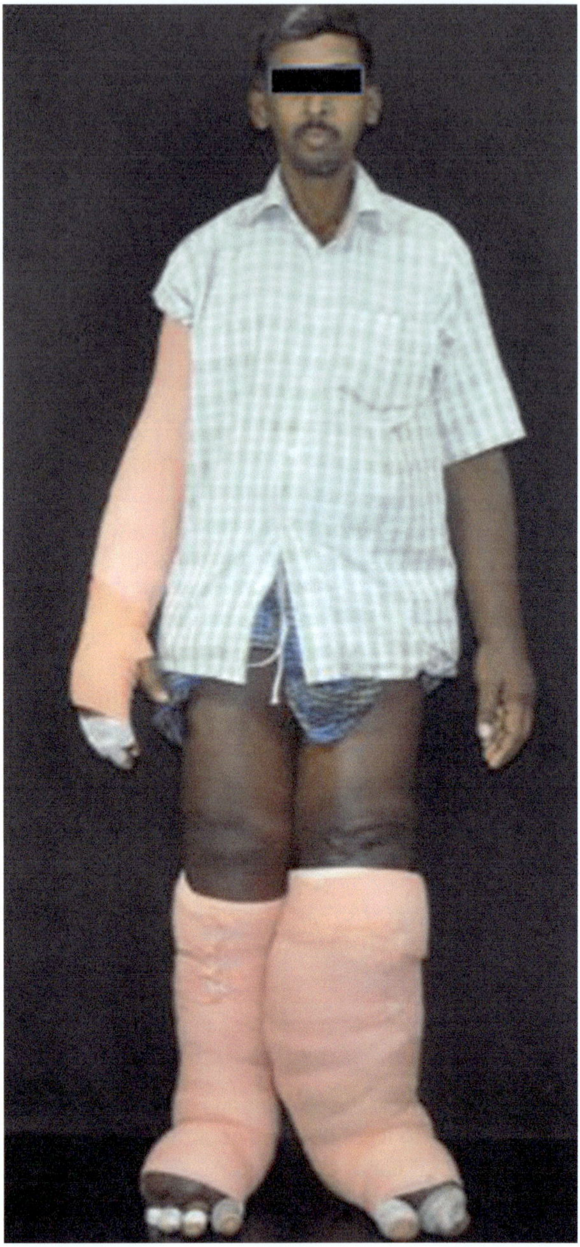

Fig. 9.34 A patient wearing compression bandages for upper and lower limbs

9.2 Conclusion

Compression therapy is an important component of integrated medicine cocktail treatment of lymphoedema (Fig. 9.35). Although invitro evidence is lacking compression therapy probably has a role in reducing lymph accumulation by increasing forward flow of lymph and exerts mechanical pressure over collagen biological stocking. This has a fundamental benefit in preventing progression of lymphoedema. Lymph contains several inflammatory mediators and it stagnation is always a risk factor for cellulitis. Compression therapy's role is therefore acknowledged by health care workers and scientists. Although compression therapy is known in India its expertise is lacking even in cities where even medical tourism is practiced to attract patients from developed countries. 15 years ago, we had to look for different kinds of compression bandaging systems available in Indian market, go to local markets in search of accessory materials. We had to include low cost compression tools for our low-income group patients. Challenges posed by patients' conditions are unique for low income settings and western compression therapy was developed had to be customised to Indian socioeconomic, tropical and low literacy environment. In this chapter we presented steps of giving compression therapy in such clinical settings and monitoring the same when patients return home.

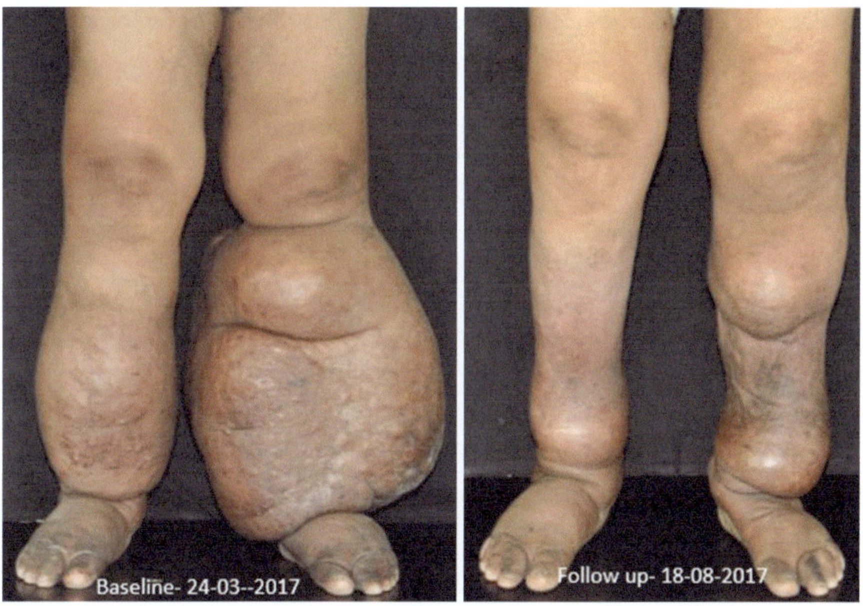

Fig. 9.35 Outcome of integrated treatment in a bilateral lower limb lymphoedema patient. Compression therapy is part of the cocktail treatment that contains low cost locally available materials with patient training for self-care

Acknowledgments We thank our patients who have given written consent to use their photographs in this chapter. Our sincere thanks to Prof. Rajgopal Mani, editor of this book for his valuable comments that helped to improve this chapter. Ms. Aneesha AR, dermatology nurse at Institute of Applied Dermatology has searched the photos from our server.

References

1. Accelerated plan for elimination of lymphatic filariasis 2018, National Vector Bore Disease Control Programme, Government of India In http://nvbdcp.gov.in/. Accessed 3 Aug 2018.
2. Indian Council for Medical Research, Public Health Foundation of India, and Institute of Health Metrics and Evaluation. India: Health of the Nation's states-The India state level Disease Burden Initiative. New Delhi, India; 2017.
3. Indian Council for Medical Research. Perspectives of Indian medicinal plants in the management of lymphatic filariasis. In: Shenoy RK, editor. . New Delhi: Indian Council for Medical Research; 2012. ISBN: 978-81-910091-1-8.
4. International Society of Lymphology. The diagnosis and treatment of peripheral lymphedema 2009. Consensus document of the international society of lymphology. Lymphology. 2009;42:51–60.
5. Foldi M, Foldi E, Kubic S. Textbook of lymphology. Munich: Elsevier; 2007.
6. Moffatt C. Compression therapy in practice. Trowbridge: Wounds UK; 2017.
7. Narahari SR, Bose KS, Aggithaya MG, Swamy GK, Ryan TJ, et al. Community level morbidity control of lymphoedema using self care and integrative treatment in two Lymphatic Filariasis endemic districts of South India – a non randomized interventional study. Trans R Soc Trop Med Hyg. 2013;107:566–77. https://doi.org/10.1093/trstmh/trt054.
8. Ryan TJ. The first commandment: oil it. An appreciation of the science underlying water and emollients for skin care. J Commun Dermatol. 2004;1:3–5.
9. The Ayurvedic formulary of India part I: department of AYUSH, government of India; 1967.
10. Narahari SR, Ryan TJ, Mahadevan PE, Bose KS, Prasanna KS. Integrated management of filarial lymphoedema for rural communities. Lymphology. 2007;40:3–13.
11. Mani R, Margolis DJ, Shukla VK, et al. Optimal use of technology in the management of chronic lower extremity wounds. Int J Low Extrem Wounds. 2016;15(2):102–19.
12. Narahari SR, Ryan TJ, Bose KS, Prasanna KS, Aggithaya GM. Integrating modern dermatology and Ayurveda in the treatment of vitiligo and lymphedema in India. Int J Dermatol. 2011;50:310–34.
13. Narahari SR, Ryan TJ, Aggithaya MG. How does yoga work in lymphedema? J Yoga Phys Ther. 2013;3:135. https://doi.org/10.4172/2157-7595.1000135.
14. Narahari S, Aggithaya MG, Ryan T. Yoga as a therapy for lymphedema. In: Telles S, Singh N, editors. Research-based applied psychophysiology. https://doi.org/10.4018/978-1-5225-2788-6.ch014. LCCN 2017010726| ISBN 9781522527886 (hardcover) | ISBN 9781522527893 (ebook) IGI Global; 2017. p. 241–62.

Chapter 10
Alternative Technological Approaches to Achieving Improved Venous Return

Mark C. Richardson

Abstract The role and importance of compression in achieving venous return is well understood and the use of multilayer compression remains the standard of care for the patient with a Venous Ulcer. However a range of alternative technologies have emerged which aim to reduce or overcome some of the disadvantages of bandaging. This chapter explores methods of pressure assessment under bandages to facilitate application of bandages and also discusses alternatives to bandaging including adjustable systems, Intermittent Pneumatic Compression (IPC) Systems and finally powered muscle stimulators. All these approaches, as the evidence supporting them develops, could offer useful alternatives to compression for a number of patient groups.

Keywords Venous ulcers · Venous disease · Compression bandages · Blood flow

10.1 Introduction

It is well accepted that an important therapeutic intervention in the successful management of the venous leg ulcer patient is the achievement of improved venous return using external compression bandages [1]. The recognised approach for delivering this therapy is that following a holistic patient assessment, a bandaging system is applied in order to achieve a graduated compression of up to 40 mmHg at the ankle and then gradually decreasing up the limb.

There are range of bandaging systems available commercially covering elastic/inelastic materials with variable number of layers. This range of products and the ability to vary application techniques to achieve lower levels of compression than the recommended 40 mmHg at ankle level mean that the clinician can select a compression system that best fits the individual patient's history, diagnosis, preferences and outcome priorities. Lower levels of compression are preferable to no compression

M. C. Richardson (✉)
University of Southampton, Southampton, UK
e-mail: M.C.Richardson@soton.ac.uk

R. Mani et al. (eds.), *Compression and Chronic Wound Management*,
https://doi.org/10.1007/978-3-030-01195-6_10

at all, so that if 40 mmHg is not achievable then working with the patient to achieve an acceptable and tolerable level of compression is a valuable process [2].

There are a number of disadvantages with existing compression systems that have led to a sustained desire to innovate and develop alternatives to current systems by clinicians, academics and companies. These disadvantages include:

- Need for clinician training in application techniques
- Limited system availability on Formularies which consequently minimise clinician choice
- Poor patient tolerance to compression or to bandage materials
- Lack of ability for patients to self-apply
- Poor conformability of bandages leading to consequent slippage
- Poor aesthetic qualities of the bandage and their materials leading to a patient reluctance or inability to maintain lifestyle (hobbies/interests)
- Patients unable to wear their own footwear with consequent effect on gait and mobility
- Patients may not be mobile e.g. in a wheelchair, and therefore a compression bandage is not appropriate.

10.2 Alternatives to Compression

It is not the purpose of this chapter to explore the variation and innovation in multilayer compression bandages (elastic/inelastic, 2–4 layer) but rather to summarise the approaches taken which take radically different but non-invasive approaches to achieving enhanced venous return.

These approaches have been categorised here as follows:

A. Adjustable compression systems.
B. Intermittent pneumatic compression systems.
C. Powered muscle stimulators.

Before considering each of these in more detail it is, however, worth commenting on one innovation which sits alongside the existing compression systems. This is the use of sub bandage pressure monitors. These devices aim to allow the clinician to assess the interfacial pressure being delivered at the bandage/skin interface to enhance the effectiveness of bandage application in achieving graduated compression. They can also be useful in the training of clinicians in application techniques. A number of commercial systems exist [3]. These include:

1. PicoPress® (Medi Group, Australia) pressure transducer which can be left under the bandage allowing for repeated measurement (Fig. 10.1).
2. Kikuhime® (Medi Group, Australia) portable sub bandage pressure monitoring device which is recommended for use for training sessions and workshops (Fig. 10.2).

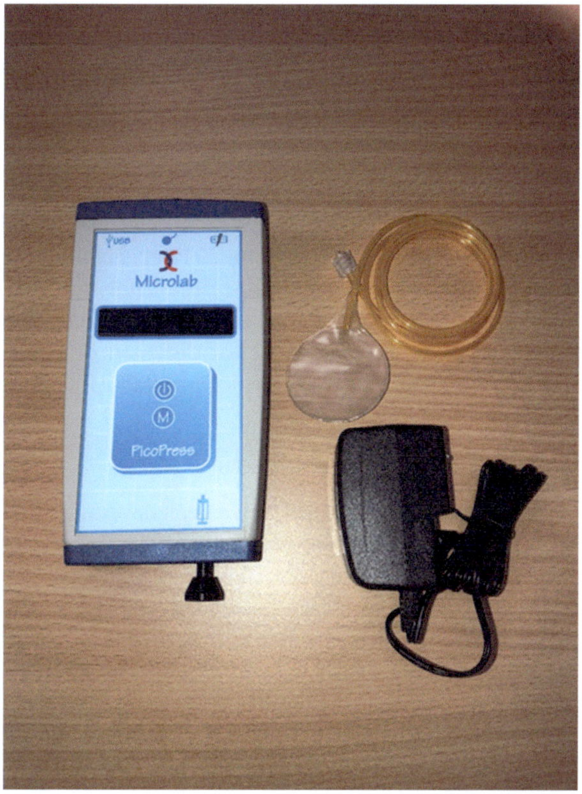

Fig. 10.1 PicoPress® (Medi Group, Australia) pressure transducer which can be left under the bandage allowing for repeated measurement

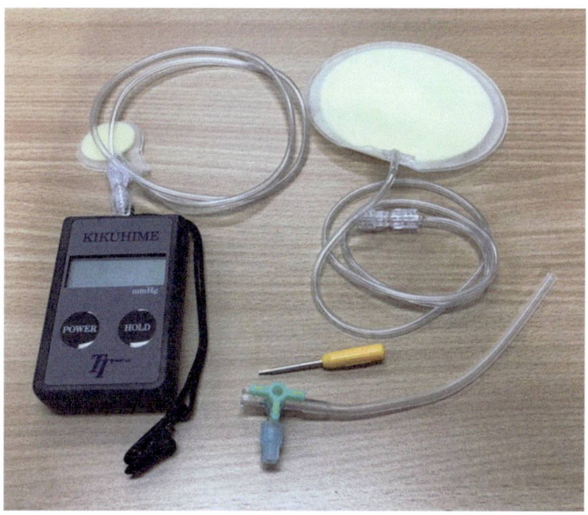

Fig. 10.2 Kikuhime® (Medi Group, Australia) portable sub bandage pressure monitoring device which is ideal for use for training sessions and workshops

3. Carolon Smart Sleeve® (Carolon, USA) This system uses an initial proprietary sleeve applied to the patient's limb and then a pressure sensor is applied across the sleeve.

A clinician's desired compression system is applied over each of these systems and then use of a separate reader allows compression pressures to be assessed whilst the compression is in place. These systems offer useful approaches to assessing the effectiveness of different compression methods as well as providing an effective approach to training and can ultimately give confidence that effective pressures are being maintained and achieved. Unfortunately the widespread constraints in financial budgets in woundcare provision globally mean that beyond their valuable use in training it may be challenging for diffusion of these devices into wider clinical practice until studies are performed to establish any improvement they allow users to achieve in clinical outcomes.

A. Adjustable compression systems

Adjustable wrap garments have been developed to overcome some of the disadvantages of existing traditional bandage systems by allowing improved ease of use and application without specialist training [4]. As a result they may more readily be applicable to self or carer based application. In addition, they provide an alternative to patients who cannot tolerate existing compression systems. These systems are rigid in nature with high stiffness leading to low resting pressure but higher pressure when the patient is active. They are available in a range of formats, applications and pressure profiles. Examples of such systems are Juxtacures (MediUK), ReadyWrap (L & R) and Jobst Farrow Wrap (BSN). Each has a system of adjustable tabs or straps using Velcro® to secure the fit once established (Fig. 10.3). Once the system is first chosen and fitted by the clinician and then subsequent visits to change dressings may be shorter leading to potential cost sav-

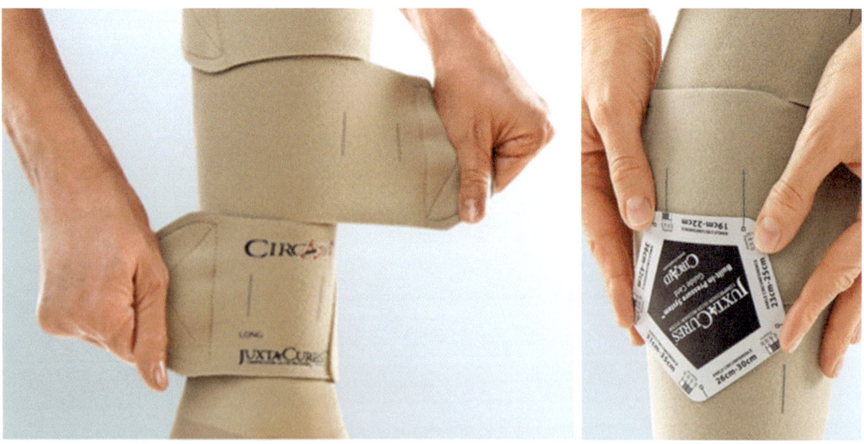

Fig. 10.3 Juxtacures (MediUK) Adjustable Compression System—this version also has an aid to help with adjustment to achieve the correct pressure depending on the limb size

ings as well as the opportunity for patient/carer application and the fact that the devices can be machine washed and re used.

These products rely not on the invention of new technology but rather on a reimagined approach to providing compression application using a series of overlapping bands secured by the use of Velcro® rather than a single circumferential wrapping approach.

B. Intermittent pneumatic compression (IPC) systems

IPC essentially uses a pump to inflate and deflate a series of bladders to effectively squeeze the limb and enhance venous return. This requires a garment/sleeve to be wrapped around the limb and connected to an external pump via a system of tubes. The electronic pump can be programmed and then deliver its therapy automatically. A Cochrane review [5] concluded that whilst the use of these systems was better than no compression at all, that there was conflicting evidence of its value relative to compression bandaging. Whilst a patient is in hospital or clinic setting then the use of these IPC systems can be under clinician control. These systems are also used to reduce the risk of DVT in at risk patients. In a home setting these systems are worth considering in order to overcome patient concordance factors which render compression or other alternatives non-viable.

The therapy cycles used in these devices have varied in reported studies but typically exert 30–40 mmHg graduated compression in 1–2 min cycle times for a variable number of hours either daily or two to three times per week. No single IPC system has been established to be superior to others. Examples of systems in use are the Synchro® system (Talley, UK) Flowtron® (Arjo Huntleigh, UK) and Kendall SCD® (Cardinal Health, USA).

Each of the IPC systems offer a range of features and benefits which may be critical in selection for particular patient groups.

A clear usability issue with these CPT systems is the need for tubing and a separate pump with the patient being immobile during therapy sessions. One technology which aims to overcome the disadvantages of the need for a bulky and potentially noisy pump is the Ventus Disc Pump System® (TTP, UK) [6]. This technology combines features of both the IPC and adjustable compression systems. The TTP system uses a proprietary disc pump whose operating system differs from that of a normal pump in that rather than changing the volume of a chamber the disc excites a high frequency standing wave in a fixed volume to deliver a pumped flow in a pump only a few centimetres in size. This pump and its power and control systems have been incorporated into an adjustable system with bladders. It aims to deliver the benefits of IPC for venous return in a lower cost more portable system. It is currently in clinical evaluation.

C. Powered muscle stimulators

An alternative approach to enhancing the venous return by the calf and foot muscle pumps is the use of neuro muscular electrostimulation (NMES). The theoretical approach is to deliver an electrical stimulation to the common peroneal nerve at the interolateral aspect of the knee joint at the fibular head. In one product (Geko®,

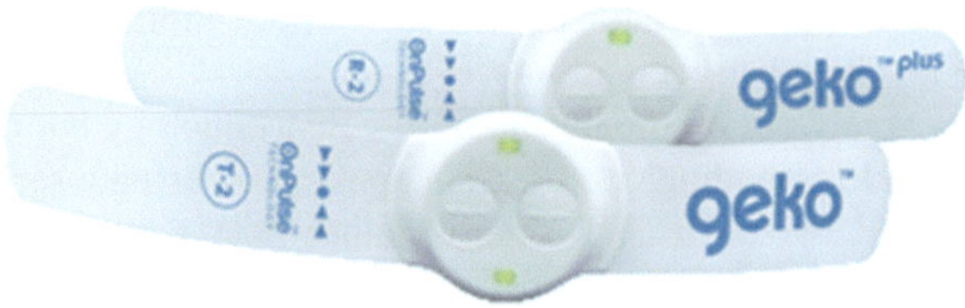

Fig. 10.4 (Geko®, Firstkind Ltd., UK) A neuro muscular electrostimulation (NMES) device. This is applied to the skin behind the knee

Firstkind Ltd., UK) this is achieved with a small adhesive wrist watch size (10 g) device applied to the skin behind the knee (Fig. 10.4).

The cyclical stimulation of the common peroneal nerve leads to the activation of muscle groups associated with the venous muscle pumps. The clinician or patient sets the stimulation level to achieve a twitching of the foot when raised from the ground. The device has been shown to increase venous, arterial and microcirculatory blood flow in the lower limb in people with chronic venous insufficiency. This device is currently undergoing clinical evaluation and a number of case studies and small studies for its use in venous ulcers have been published [7].

10.3 Conclusion

A number of alternative approaches to bandaging for the delivery of improved venous return are available or in development. Each of these aims to address one or more of the current disadvantages or problems with existing systems described in the introduction. Importantly, each will and does offer a potential alternative for patients allowing them to better achieve their treatment goals.

References

1. Harding K, Dowsett C, Flas L, et al. Simplifying venous leg ulcer management: consensus recommendations. Wounds International. 2015. https://tinyurl.com/jrxfcrj. Accessed 10 Jun 2018.
2. Franks P, Barker J, Collier M, et al. Management of patients with venous leg ulcers: challenges and current best practice. J Wound Care. 2016;25(Suppl 6):S1–S67. http://ewma.org/?id=219. Accessed 10 Jun 2018
3. Partsch H, Mosti G. Comparison of three portable instruments to measure compression pressure. Int Angiol. 2010;29(5):426–30.
4. Mahoney K, Ovens L, Harris E, et al. A proven alternative to compression bandaging: clinical review of Juxtacures. J Wound Care. 2017;26(4 Suppl 1):S1–23.
5. Nelson EA, Hillman A, Thomas K. Intermittent pneumatic compression for treating venous leg ulcers. Cochrane Database Syst Rev. 2014;5:CD001899.
6. https://tinyurl.com/y93m8kz3. Accessed 10 Jun 2018.
7. Harris C, Loney A, Brooke J, et al. Refractory venous leg ulcers: observational evaluation of innovative new technology. Int Wound J. 2017;14(6):1100–7.

Chapter 11
Advances in Devices that Offer Lower Limb Compression

Ravi Mani, Kittipan Rerkasem, and Raj Mani

Abstract The theme of this book is compression which is a mainstay of treatment for venous leg ulcers. In other parts of this book, there are descriptions of how elasticated garments are used, the evidence of success to heal wounds as well as the shortcomings of this technique that beg questions of how compression may be delivered using other methods. These include surgery to treat incompetence in the superficial veins, advances on traditional bandages and intermittent pneumatic compression (IPC). Initially IPC devices were recommended to treat lymphoedema, later these were used to treat venous conditions. The different uses, range of treatment times were systematically reviewed and reported to be of low level of confidence. Recent developments in devices have been reviewed in this chapter which especially complements Chap. 10 by Mark Richardson that deals with techniques of improving bandaging systems.

Keywords Intermittent compression · Sequential contraction compression · Calf compression · Wound healing

Flowtron™ (Arjo Huntleigh, UK) the first of intermittent pneumatic compression (IPC) devices to be used to manage limb swelling, is described in another chapter in

R. Mani
Brighton and Sussex Medical School, University of Brighton, Brighton, UK

K. Rerkasem
Department of Surgery, NCD Centre of Excellence, Chiang Mai University, Chiang Mai, Thailand

Faculty of Medicine, Chiang Mai University, Chiang Mai, Thailand

R. Mani (✉)
Academic Division of Human Health and Development, Faculty of Medicine, University of Southampton, Southampton, UK

Faculty of Medicine, Chiang Mai University, Chiang Mai, Thailand

Shanghai Jiao Tong University School of Medicine, Shanghai, China
e-mail: rm1@soton.ac.uk

R. Mani et al. (eds.), *Compression and Chronic Wound Management*,
https://doi.org/10.1007/978-3-030-01195-6_11

this book. It is described how using either a single or more bladders and an air pump designed to quickly inflate/deflate, limb swelling can be managed. Clearly this can benefit treatment of lymphoedema and venous leg ulcers both of which are therapeutic challenges whose standardised clinical management is based on compression and wound care as required [1]. Since IPC was first described, sequential contraction compression devices (SCCD) have been reported. Recent innovations include the Flow Ox™(Otivio Olso, Norway) that works on a modified IPC method as well as Flow Aid (FA)™ (FlowAid Technologies, New York) that is a SCCD and Geko™(FirstKind Medical): the latter two use electrical stimulation to activate muscular contractions.

Early attempts to treat venous leg ulcers using the Flowtron™(Arjo Huntleigh, UK) technique were reported despite the evidence being from different study types (see Table 11.1) [2, 3–17]. The early Flowtron™ devices (in the 1980s) were typically shaped like a cylinder that could be inflated with a limb inside. There were practical difficulties in using these devices and clinical reports to use this device had differing aims, outcome measures and application times. Nonetheless it is clear that controlled mechanical pressure around limb can and does promote venous blood flow as presented in clear review of the physics of the technique [18]. Very recently, Flow Ox™ (Otivio, Oslo, Norway) developed an innovation that uses a modified IPC technique to benefit both macro and micro vascular supply in foot skin and lower limb flow. The Flow Ox™ device is essentially a sealed chamber that connects to an air pump (see Fig. 11.1). In use, a patient would position the lower limb needing treatment in the chamber, resting the foot on the rocker bottom. The top of the chamber is sealed using a flexible cuff to form an air tight compartment before the it (the chamber) is connected to the air pump within the control unit. The seal (flexible cuff) is washable in water, it has a life time of months. Air pressure within the chamber is varied between −40 mmHg below atmosphere and atmospheric pressure. Time of variation can be altered to suit needs: a setting commonly used is 10 s at −40 mmHg and 7 s at atmospheric pressure.

Using these on a group of patients with peripheral arterial disease ($N = 20$, mean age 75 years, statistically significant increases over baseline values were reported in peak arterial flow 46% $p < 0.001$, peak skin blood flow or perfusion 89% $p < 0.001$ while mean blood flow velocity increased by 12% (6.7–75. cm/s) $p = 0.03$ [19]. It is postulated that the device works by modulating the air chamber pressures *without* triggering the arterio-venous reflex. The device has been used to treat chronic lower extremity wounds including a group of patients with spinal cord injury and lower extremity wounds [20]. This cohort included paraplegic and tetraplegic patients. A randomised, single centre, observed-blinded cross over study was done on patients ($N = 9$, age 57 years IQR 52–66 years) with chronic wounds duration 52 weeks (IQR 12–82 weeks). Flow Ox™ plus standardised care was compared against stan-

Table 11.1 Selected reports of Intermittent Pneumatic Compression (IPC) use

Name (year)	Type of study Length of study	*N*=	1. Independent variables 2. Patient group 3. IPC device 4. IPC regime	Results
Alpagut (2005)	RCT 3 months	235	1. IPC + compression therapy vs. control (leg elevation + elastic compression stockings) 2. Patients with post-thrombotic syndrome venous leg ulcers (VLU) 3. Device: Flowtron Plus AC 20002 (Huntleigh Healthcare, UK) 4. Regime: 1 h OD max pressure 70 mmHg	Response to therapy IPC: 100% (76/76) Control: 93.7% (149/159) Time to healing IPC: 20 days (15–35 days) Control: 3 months (20 days–5 months) Return to activity IPC: 7 days Control: 25 days
Alvarez (2012)	RCT 12 months	52	1. IPC + compression bandaging vs. control (compression bandaging alone) 2. Patients with VLU and secondary lymphoedema 3. Device: Sequential Circulator Model 2004 (BioCompression Inc., USA) 4. Regime: 1 h BD 40–50 mmHg	Median time to wound closure by 9 months IPC: 141 days Control: 211 days ($p = 0.031$) Ulcer healing rate (mm/day) IPC: 2.3 mm ±0.08 Control: 1.1 ± 0.04 ($p < 0.05$) Reduction in leg oedema (not significant) IPC: 19.1% Control: 12.0%
Coleridge smith (1989)	RCT 3 months or to healing	45	1. IPC + compression stockings vs. control (compression stockings alone) 2. Patients with VLU 3. Device not stated 4. Regime: Up to 4 h per day, 30–40 mmHg	Number of ulcers healed IPC: 10/21 (48%) Control: 1/24 (4%) Median reduction in area IPC: 19.8%/week Control: 2.1%/week

(continued)

Table 11.1 (continued)

Name (year)	Type of study Length of study	*N*=	1. Independent variables 2. Patient group 3. IPC device 4. IPC regime	Results
Dolibog (2013)	Randomised pilot study 15 days	70	1. IPC vs. compression stockings vs. short-stretch bandages 2. Patients with unilateral VLUs and chronic venous insufficiency 3. Device: Flowtron Hydroven 12 System device (Huntleigh Healthcare, UK) 4. Regime: 1 h OD, 60 mmHg at ankle and 40 mmHg at groin.	Average wound size decrease in patients w/ superficial venous reflux IPC: 9.91 cm^2, 20.12–10.21 cm^2 Stockings: 9.00 cm^2, 19.45–10.45 cm^2 Bandages: 8.77 cm^2, 17.23–8.46 cm^2 Average wound size decrease in patients w/ superficial + deep venous reflux IPC: 9.33 cm^2, 19.35–10.02 cm^2 Stockings: 5.05 cm^2, 25.09–20.04 cm^2 Bandages: 2.78 cm^2, 24.67–21.89 cm^2 Proportion of completely healed ulcers in patients with superficial venous reflux after 15 days IPC: 25% Stockings: 27% Bandages: 10%
Grieveson (2003)	Randomised trial	27	1. IPC vs. control (elevation of legs) 2. Patients with chronic venous insufficiency 3. Device: Flowpac pump (Huntleigh Healthcare Ltd, UK) 4. IPC at variety of pressures 30–70 mmHg—Full strategy not stated	Highest mean reduction in limb volume at 40 mmHg Significant results at 30 mmHg Lower pressures + shorter inflation/deflation times more efficient than higher pressures + long inflation/deflation times
Hazarika (1981)	Case series 44 weeks	21	1. IPC vs. control (compression bandaging alone) 2. Patients with VLU 3. Device: Flowtron (Huntleigh Healthcare, UK) 4. Regime: 2–3 h OD, 30–80 mmHg	Number of improved ulcers IPC: 71.4% (5/7) Control: 8.3% (1/12)

Table 11.1 (continued)

Name (year)	Type of study Length of study	$N=$	1. Independent variables 2. Patient group 3. IPC device 4. IPC regime	Results
Kumar (2002)	RCT 4 months	47	1. IPC + 4-layer bandaging vs. control (4-layer compression) 2. Patients with VLU 3. Device: Not stated 4. Regime: Used for 1 h BD	Number of ulcers healed IPC: 20/23 ulcers (87%) Control: 23/25 healed (92%)
McCulloch (1994)	RCT 6 months	22	1. IPC + standard compression (Unna boot) vs. control (Unna boot) 2. Patients with VLU 3. Device: Not stated 4. Regime: Twice weekly for 1 h each session at 55 mmHg	Number of ulcers healed IPC 12/12 (100%) Control 8/10 (80%) Mean healing rate (cm2/day) IPC 0.15 cm^2/day Control 0.08 cm^2/day ($p = 0.05$)
Mulder (1990)	Cohort study 1 year	10	1. IPC vs. Unna boot 2. Patients with VLU 3. Device: not stated (from Kendall Healthcare, UK) 4. Regime: IPC used OD for 1 h in morning then 2 h in evening	All patients healed 1 patient healed by 4 months ($p < 0.01$)
Nikolovska (2002)	RCT 6 months	80	The efficacy of intermittent pneuma tic compression in the treatment of venous leg ulcers 1. IPC vs. control 2. Patients with VLU 3. Device: not stated 4. Regime: IPC used for 1 h OD for 5 days a week, 40–50 mmHg	Number of ulcers healed IPC: 25/40 (62.5%) Control: 11/40 (27.5%)
Nikolovska (2005)	Randomised trial 6 months/until ulcer completely healed	104	1. Rapid vs. slow IPC 2. Patients with VLU 3. Device: not stated 4. Rapid vs. slow IPC, specific regimes not stated	Complete ulcer healing Rapid IPC 45/52 (86.5%) Slow IPC 32/52 (61.5%) Mean healing rate/day Rapid IPC 0.09 cm^2/day Slow IPC 0.04 cm^2/day ($P = 0.0002$)

(continued)

Table 11.1 (continued)

Name (year)	Type of study Length of study	*N*=	1. Independent variables 2. Patient group 3. IPC device 4. IPC regime	Results
Pekenmaki (1987)	Open clinical trial	8	1. IPC + compression therapy vs. control (compression therapy alone) in post-thrombotic leg ulcers 2. Patients with post-thrombotic syndrome VLU 3. Device: not stated 4. Regime: not stated	IPC + conservative treatment shortened ulcer healing time vs. conservative treatment alone
Rowland (2000)	RCT 6 months	16	1. IPC vs. control (compression therapy using Septopress bandaging) 2. Patients with VLU 3. Device: Flowtron (Huntleigh Healthcare, Australia) 4. Regime: IPC used for 1 h BD (morning + evening)	Ulcer size No significant difference Lower limb volume No significant difference
Schuler (1996)	RCT 6 months	54	1. IPC + elasticated stockings graduated compression stockings vs. control (Unna boot) 2. Patients with VLU 3. Device: HomeRx (Kendall Healthcare, UK) 4. Regime: IPC applied for 1 h each morning and 2 h each evening (40–50 mmHg)	Complete ulcer healing: IPC: 20/28 (71%) Control: 15/25 (60%) Healing rates IPC: 76% Control: 64% – **not significant**
Smith (1990)	RCT 3 months	45	1. IPC + compression stockings vs. control (compression stockings alone) 2. Patients with VLU 3. Device: not stated (provided by Kendall Healthcare, UK) 4. Device: IPC applied for 4 h a day, between 40 and 50 mmHg	Number of VLU healed IPC: 10/21 47.6% Control: 1/23 4.3% ($P = 0$) Median healing rate (area/week) IPC: 19.8% Control: 2.1% ($p = 0.046$)

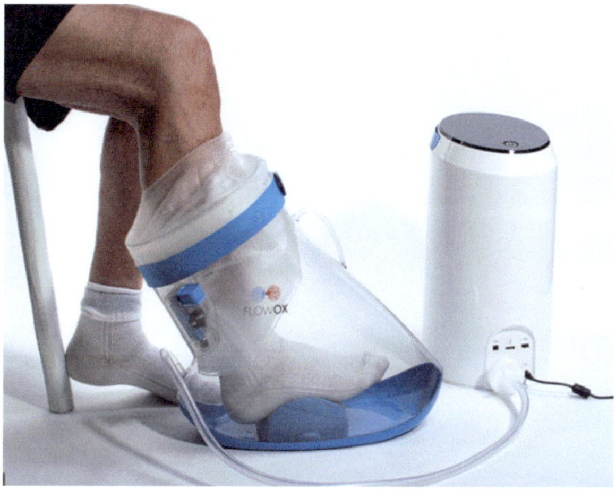

Fig. 11.1 Shows a subject with his foot resting on the rocker sole of the Flow Ox™ air chamber. The controller housing the air pump is the cylindrical device with a flexible hose to connect to the air chamber. The seal (or flexible cuff) is washable. Used with Permission of Otivio™ (Otivio, Olso, Norway)

dard care alone over 8 weeks. Flow Ox was™ used for 2 h in patients' homes, PWAT (a validated scoring system) was used to assess wound changes.

This pilot study aimed to determine patient compliance and to explore wound healing potential. It reported 90% compliance to Flow Ox™ use, additionally there was a significant trend in wound healing in 4/4 patients while on Flow Ox™ plus standard care. To truly appreciate these findings, one must consider the study group who were paraplegic or tetraplegics a cohort with limited mobility, often have functional venous disease and on whom, compression bandaging is very difficult to use. A few clinical images of wounds are shown in Fig. 11.2.

11.1 Change in Contraction Patterns

A sequential contraction compression device (SCCD) compresses calf muscles in sausage like fashion: top and bottom squeezed while middle is held open: this forces venous flow out of bottom (filling the middle) and top (towards the thigh) while the middle segment fills but neither expels nor allows downward flow. Then the reverse follows with top and bottom segments open while middle is closed forcing flow out of the middle segment but not permitting any inflow at the bottom and no reflux from the top segment. The FlowAid FA100 Sequential Continuous Contraction Device (SCCD) electrically stimulates specific groups of calf muscles. These contractions, which run from distal to proximal along the leg, cause a peristaltic wave of compressions. This compresses the deep veins, causing venous outflow and, secondarily, arterial inflow.

The FlowAid FA100 SCCD system (FlowAid Medical Technologies Corporation, NY, USA) is a handheld unit using four electrodes to deliver electrical currents at three pre-set contraction frequencies to suit such different conditions as Venous, Arterial, Lymphoedema, and Diabetic Neuropathy. It is recommended that the

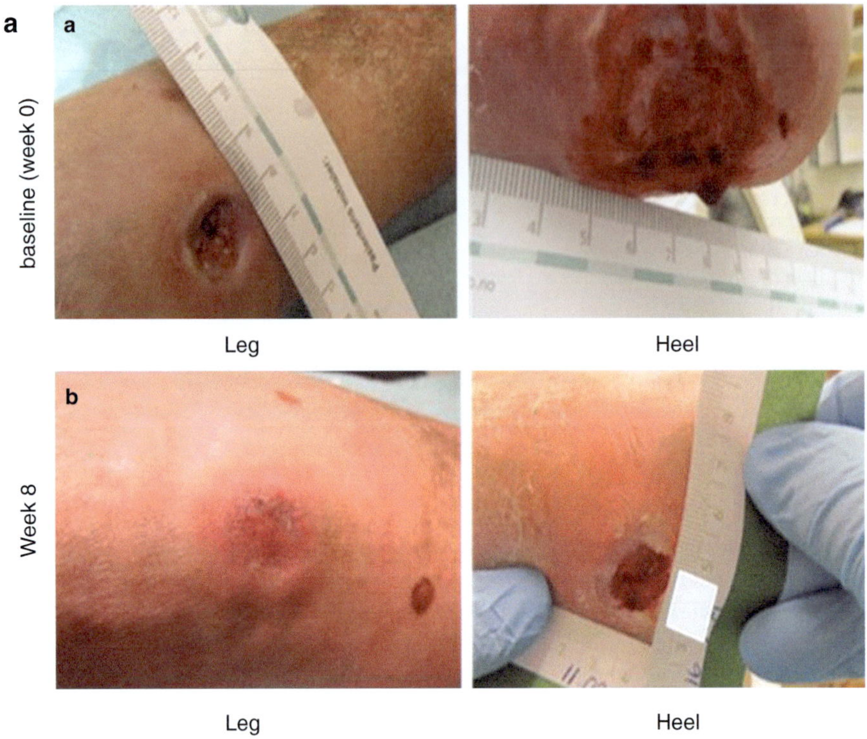

Fig. 11.2 (**a**) Shows four images of two lower extremity chronic wounds both treated with Flow Ox™ for 8 weeks. *A* is the status at baseline and B after 8 weeks treatment with Flow Ox™ in the study. Images on the Left of are of a chronic wound on the medial aspect of the leg while those on the *Right* show a chronic wound on a heel. Notice the Leg *A* wound is deep with rounded edges while the same wound in *B* below, is mostly fully covered with epithelium. The wound the heel on (Right) is extensive as can be seen in *A*. After treatment with Flow Ox™ improvement in size as well as the quality surrounding skin may be observed in *B*. Wounds on heels are difficult to manage. From Sundby ØH, Høiseth LO, Mathiesen I et al. The acute effects of lower limb intermittent negative pressure on foot macro and microcirculation in patients with peripheral arterial disease. PLOSONE https://doi.org/10.1371/jounral.pone.017900 June 2017. Reproduced with permission https://physoc.onlinelibrary.wiley.com/hub/journal/2051817x/about/permissions. (**b**) presents a chronic wound on the forefoot treated with Flow Ox. The patient is diabetic with renal failure. On account of the open wound, he was not offered a transplant. Using the Flow Ox device, resulted in improvement over 26 weeks associated with an increase in ABI (ankle brachial pressure index) in the treated leg. This a classic example of improved macro and microvascular flow resulting from use of Flow Ox. Used with Permission from Otivio, Oslo, Norway

b

WOUND HEALING IN A PATIENT WITH DIABETES AND RENAL FAILURE TREATED WITH FLOW OX™ (OTIVIO, OSLO, NORWAY

Male 45 years old
- 7 year old wound
- Not offered kidney transplant due to open wound
- Significant long term improved blood flow
- Now on the transplant list for a new kidney

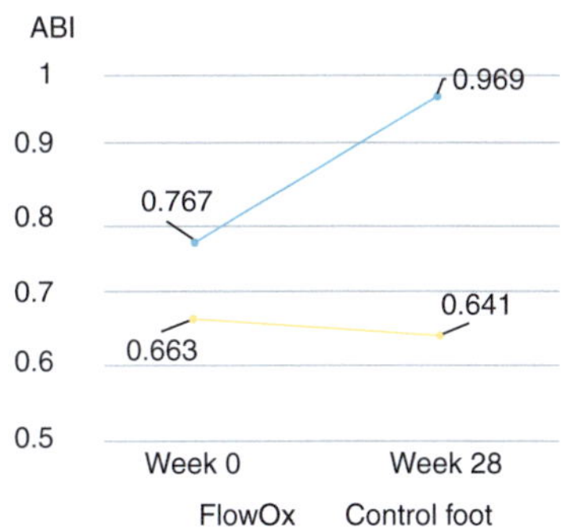

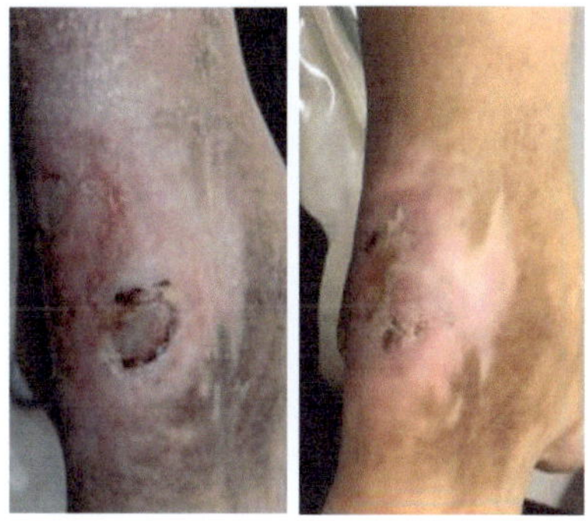

Fig. 11.2 (continued)

device be used for 1.5 h both in the morning and in the evening for optimal performance. Patients may choose a comfortable resting position or be ambulant when the device is in operation. Figure 11.3 shows four electrodes placed on the lower leg over the calf muscles using the FA100 SCCD. The handheld unit houses the controller and the rechargeable power supply.

An evaluation of the FA100 SCCD device to determine effects on popliteal vein blood flow in volunteers (n = 11, 22 limbs (age 25–45 years)) showed that FA100 increases flow in the popliteal vein 317% and active dorsi flexion of the foot 437% compared to the passive resting sitting position [21]. Gimmelreich [22] studied the effect of FA100 SCCD on patients with bilateral chronic venous insufficiency (CVI) to determine the effects of reducing afterload by measuring ankle and calf circumference on patients. Patients with CVI (N = 15) who were being treated with compression to manage their conditions were included. Patients applied FA100 SCCD following their prescribed elasticated stocking or IPC compression. Initially all subjects were treated and had their ankle and calf circumferences measured at baseline and following 2 h FA100 SCCD treatment. Patients on FA100 SCCD plus compression group continued

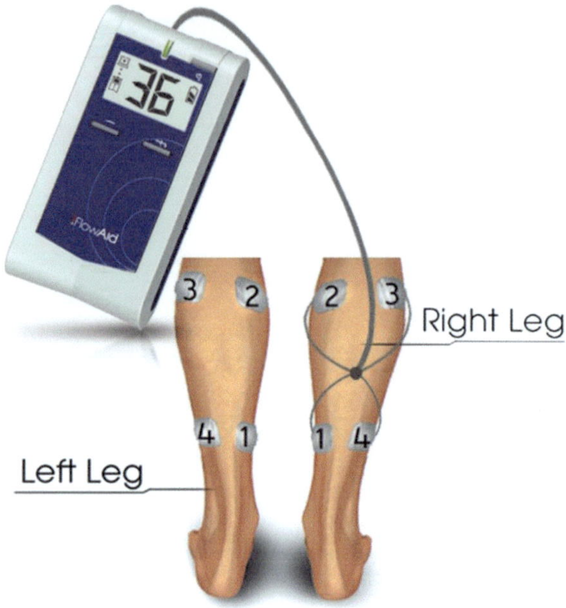

Fig. 11.3 Shows electrodes in situ on a leg using the FA device. The palm top size case houses the controller and the rechargeable power supply for the unit. Used with permission from Flow Aid (Medical Technology, USA)

to use the SCCD treatment for 2 h twice daily for 30 days while others were on compression garments before returning to the clinic for ankle and calf measurements.

In the test limb after 30 days, there were statistically significant reductions in circumference at ankle (21.9%, $p < 0.05$) and calf (19.5%, $p < 0.01$) respectively. Statistically significant trends were evident in the calf even after 2 h of FA100 use. By comparison, using standard compression (elasticated stocking or IPC) there were no significant changes versus the baseline except at the ankle at 30 days, where there was a reduction of 7.23% ($p < 0.05$). This is a very useful objective measure of improved venous outflow activity and helpful surrogate measure of wound healing. Complete compression cycles (distal to proximal) of the FA100 SCCD are far higher than any of the IPC devices in current use.

Two different chronic wounds that responded well to FA100 SCCD use are shown in Fig. 11.4a–d.

11.2 GEKO™ (FirstKind)

The Geko™ device uses neuro-electrical stimulation as described in Chap. 10. The device is small and may be neatly position on the popliteal nerve in the space behind the knee as shown in Fig. 10.4. In use, the level of stimulation current is adjusted to

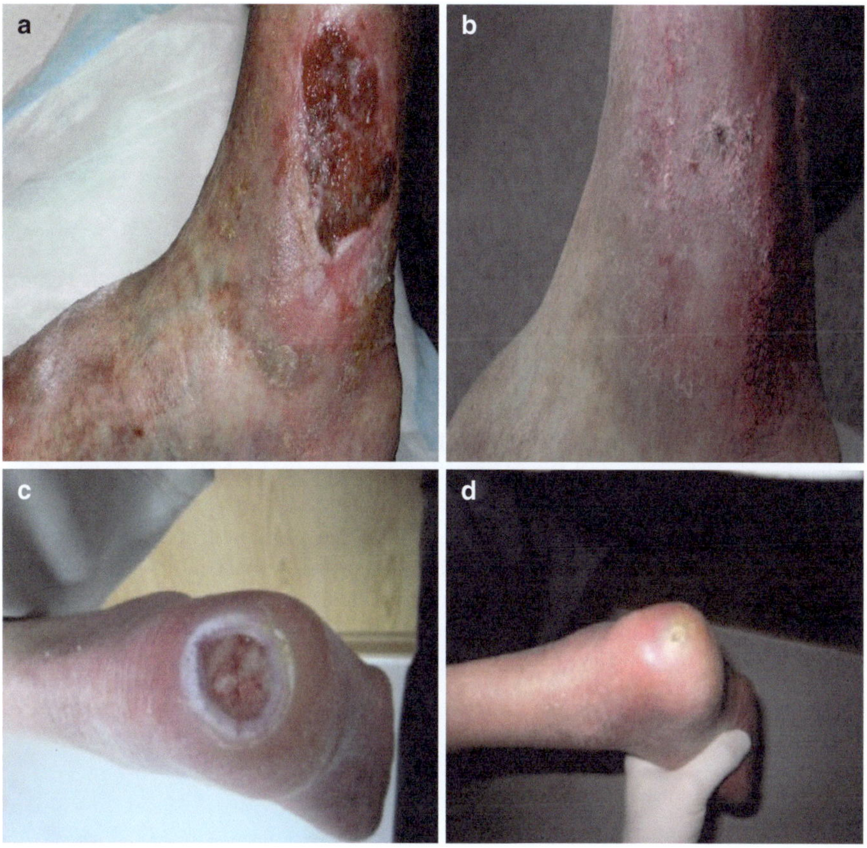

Fig. 11.4 (**a**, **b**) show a chronic venous leg ulcer in the malleolar region of the leg that responded to FA treatment for 4 weeks. This wound was circumferential. Reproduced with Permission from FlowAid Medical Technologies, New York. (**c** (left) and **d** (right)) show healing in a chronic wound on the heel of a 72 year old male that are difficult to treat with success. The wound started as a war injury and was very painful. Use of FA 100 3 h daily resulted in dramatic healing and much decreased pain. Reproduced with Permission from FlowAid Medical Technologies, New York

obtain muscle movements which in turn stimulates venous outflow and arterial inflow. The device is battery powered and is a single use device.

The aim of using the GEKO is to mimic walking: by stimulating the peroneal nerve, muscle groups in the calf are stimulated which in turn increases venous blood flow which has potential to benefit some patients at risk of venous thromboembolism. NICE has "recommended GEKO™ use in patients with a high risk of venous thromboembolism when other mechanical/pharmacological methods of prophylaxis are impractical or contraindicated with the National Health Service in England" [23]. Flowtron™ (Arjo Huntleigh, UK) is also recommended for use to prevent venous thromboembolism™ especially in maternity hospitals in the UK. Returning to basics, the property to improve venous outflow is a significant step towards better wound health.

11.3 Conclusion

External calf compression using pneumatic and electro-stimulation permit venous outflow to increase which in turn, benefits reduction of oedema. And since reduction of oedema benefits wound healing, this benefits tissue health. There is evidence both laboratory based and from the clinic that Flow Ox™ and Flow (FA) devices have the capacity to improve wound healing.

The study using FlowAid by Gemmerlich [22] et al. measured changes in ankle and calf circumference and found significant reductions in both parameters. This augers well for the device and the use of calf and ankle circumference as a surrogate measure of wound healing. The Flow Ox™ device promoted healing in patients with spinal lesions: every patient who needs compression must get it—the universal question is how to deliver it? These innovative devices have shown their promise. Both Flow Aid (FA) and Flow Ox™ studies have shown high patient compliance. There is a great deal to come from these devices to benefit patients with chronic wounds and limb swelling.

References

1. Mani R, Margolis D, Shukla VK, et al. Optimal use of technology to manage chronic lower extremity wounds a consensus document. Int J Low Extrem Wounds. 2016;15(2):102–19.
2. Nelson EA, Hillman A, Thomas K. Intermittent pneumatic compression for treating venous leg ulcers. Cochrane Databas Syt Rev. 2014;(5):CD001899. https://doi.org/10.1002/14651858.CD001899.pub4.
3. Alpagut U, Dayioglu E. Importance and advantages of intermittent external pneumatic compression therapy in venous stasis ulceration. Angiology. 2005;56(1):19–23.
4. Alvarez O, Wendelken M, Markowitz L, Parker R, Comfort C. Effectiveness of intermittent pneumatic compression for the treatment of venous ulcers in subjects with secondary (acquired) lymphedema. Vein. 2012;5(1):32–4.
5. Coleridge Smith PD, Sarin SA, Wilson LAA, Scurr JH. Intermittent pneumatic compression improves venous ulcer healing. Phlebologie '89. Paris: John Libbey Eurotext; 1989. p. 1146–8.
6. Dolibog P, Franek A, Taradaj J, Polak A, Dolibog P, Blaszczak E, et al. A randomized, controlled clinical pilot study comparing three types of compression therapy to treat venous leg ulcers in patients with superficial and/or segmental deep venous reflux. Ostomy Wound Manage. 2013;59(8):22–30.
7. Grieveson S. Intermittent pneumatic compression pump settings for the optimum reduction of oedema. J Tissue Viability. 2003;13(3):98–100.
8. Hazarika EZ. Chronic leg ulcers. The effect of pneumatic intermittent compression. Practitioner. 1981;225:189–92.

9. Kumar S, Samraj K, Nirujogi V, Budnik J, Walker MA. Intermittent pneumatic compression as an adjuvant therapy in venousulcer disease. J Tissue Viability. 2002;12(2):42–4.
10. McCulloch JM, Marler KC, Neal MB, Phifer TJ. Intermittent pneumatic compression improves venous ulcer healing. Adv Wound Care. 1994;7(4):22–4. 26
11. Mulder G. Study of sequential compression therapy in the treatment of non-healing chronic venous ulcers. Wounds. 1990;2:111–5.
12. Nikolovska S, Pavlova LJ, Petrova N, Gocev G. The efficacy of intermittent pneumatic compression in the treatment of venous leg ulcers. Mac Med Rev. 2002;5:56–9.
13. Nikolovska S, Arsovski A, Damevska K, Gocev G, Pavlova L. Evaluation of two different intermittent pneumatic compression cycle settings in the healing of venous ulcers: a randomized trial. Med Sci Monit. 2005;11(7):CR337–43.
14. Pekanmaki K, Kolari PJ, Kiistala U. Intermittent pneumatic compression treatment for post-thrombotic leg ulcers. Clin Exp Dermatol. 1987;12:350–3.
15. Rowland J. Intermittent pump versus compression bandages in the treatment of venous leg ulcers. Aust N Z J Surg. 2000;70(2):110–3.
16. Schuler JJ, Maibenco T, Megerman J, Ware M, Montalvo J. Treatment of chronic venous ulcers using sequential gradient intermittent pneumatic compression. Phlebology. 1996;11(3):111–6.
17. Smith PC, Sarin S, Hasty J, Scurr JH. Sequential gradient pneumatic compression enhances venous ulcer healing: a randomized trial. Surgery. 1990;108(5):871–5.
18. Morris RJ, Woodcock JP. Evidence-based compression prevention of stasis and deep vein thrombosis. Ann Surg. 2004;239(2):162–71. https://doi.org/10.1097/01.sla.0000109.77.194.66.
19. Sundby ØH, Høiseth LO, Mathiesen I, et al. The acute effects of lower limb intermittent negative pressure on foot macro and microcirculation in patients with peripheral arterial disease. PLoS One. 2017;12(6):e0179001. https://doi.org/10.1371/jounral.pone.0179001.
20. Sundby ØH, Irgrens I, Høiseth LO, Mathiesen I, et al. Intermittent mild negative pressure applied to the lower limb in patients with spinal cord injury and chronic lower limb ulcers: a cross over pilot study. Spinal Cord. 2018;56(4):372–81. https://doi.org/10.1038/S41393.018-0030-4.
21. Shashar D, Rosenblaum J, Miller M, Heldingberg E, Tamir J. Evaluation of a novel compressive device on popliteal venous blood flow. Angiology. 2016;4:178. https://doi.org/10.4172/2329-9495.1000178.
22. Gemmelreich D, Karsilnov V, Litman V, Rosenblaum J. Sequential contraction compression devices reduce leg circumference in patients with chronic venous insufficiency. J Vasc Med Sur. 2016;4:4. https://doi.org/10.4172/2329-6925.1000283.
23. Summers JA, Clinch J, Radhakrishnan M, et al. The geko™ electro-stimulation device for venous thromboembolism prophylaxis: a NICE medical technology guidance. Appl Health Econ Health Policy. 2015;13(2):135–247. https://doi.org/10.1007/s40258-014-0139-0.

Chapter 12
Flap Surgery and Compression Therapy

Joon Pio(Jp) Hong and Hyunsuk Peter Suh

Abstract Although early ambulation is critical to minimize postoperative morbidity and improve the quality of life after the flap surgery, many surgeons hesitate to dangle or tell the patient to ambulate due to the concern of compression and obstruction of the flap pedicle in the early recovery phase. In this chapter, the personal experience regarding the flap compression in extremities with customized pressure garments to prevent swelling and venous congestion after perforator-based flap to reconstruct the soft tissue defect will be described.

Keywords Perforator flap · Compression · Dangling

12.1 Introduction

Free flap surgery or perforator flap based surgery including propeller flap and keystone flap now become a routine surgical method and procedure for covering the soft tissue defect of a traumatized lower extremity or after cancer ablation surgery. Soft tissue flap can prevent major amputation and can minimize the morbidity after trauma or cancer ablative surgery or diabetic ulcer management. Soft tissue flap, especially skin perforator flap is superior to split thickness skin graft or full-thickness skin graft in its thickness and bulkiness. The thickness of the flap adds the durability against the pressure and shearing, and prevent the flap from getting ulcerated during the ambulation. That is the reason many of the flap surgeries are used to cover the defect on lower extremities although it is technically difficult than the split or full-thickness skin graft.

After flap coverage, when a patient starts ambulation in the early recovery phase, there is a high probability that the reconstructed flap and the limb will have swelling and transient congestion because of the gravity and mobilization [1, 2],

J. P. Hong (✉) · H. P. Suh
Department of Plastic and Reconstructive Surgery, Asan Medical Center, University of Ulsan College of Medicine, Seoul, South Korea
e-mail: joonphong@amc.seoul.kr

R. Mani et al. (eds.), *Compression and Chronic Wound Management*,
https://doi.org/10.1007/978-3-030-01195-6_12

although the dangling the limb can increase the oxygenation and hemoglobin concentration within the flap [3]. The reason of swelling is because the connection of the flap, through which the fluid and the perfusion can be transferred, is only based on the anastomosed vessel or the pedicle in the early phase and the inosculation or the neovascularization from the flap to the surrounding tissue or the opposite is not well established yet. Especially the veins within the flap do not have any aid from the muscle pumping and will have high venous pressure compare to the surrounding cutaneous veins or the deep veins while it is on the dependent position.

These increased venous pressure and hydrostatic pressure puts a strain on the flap. Not only causing massive swelling and wound dehiscence, it can block the venous outflow from the flap and cause venous thrombosis and flap necrosis [4, 5].

So, before letting the patients to lower the leg and walk with their reconstructed limb, challenging the flap and limb has been considered by most of the surgeons. There are several studies regarding the microcirculatory basis of challenging. The common challenging procedure is dangling the limb with compression for few days before ambulation. By wrapping the flap, venous return from the soft tissue flap and the venolymphatic flow in improved [1, 2, 4, 6].

Even though early compression after perforator-based flap surgery is an obvious benefit, vascular pedicle compression of the perforator-based flap was the main concern and worry. If the compression pressure exceeds the arterial pressure of the transferred flap, flap perfusion is endangered and if the compression pressure is not enough there will be the minimal effect of compression.

In this chapter, we will discuss regarding our postoperative compression protocol based on the study about the flow of the perforator pedicle after compression and show the safety of early flap compression.

12.2 A Physiological Difference Base on the Surgical Methods of Perforator Based Flaps

12.2.1 Propeller Flap

In the recent decade, propeller flap has become one of the flap of choice for soft tissue defect coverage [7]. As the circulation of a propeller flap is based on the single perforator, the length of which is usually limited. As the flap is rotated on this perforator, there is a chance of excessive tension or the torsion and kinking of the pedicle. Although the surgical technique is important and all the kinking and tension should be eliminated intraoperatively, excessive tension can newly develop after the surgery because of the traction or additional tension on the margin during the position change [8].

12.2.2 *Free Perforator Flap*

As the donor pedicle of the free flap can be harvest after measuring the distance from the recipient pedicle to the defect, tension on the pedicle and anastomosis is less common than propeller flap and accordingly, partial flap necrosis is significantly less [9]. After suturing the flap margin, the flap can still compress the pedicle especially if there is a tension on the flap margin or the pedicle lies over the bony prominence. When the pedicle should travel in between the tendons or through the subcutaneous tunnel, there is a high possibility of excessive compression or occlusion on the certain point of the vascular pedicle, which might endanger the flap perfusion and lead to flap failure.

12.3 Compression Protocol

An early compression protocol is recommended to all resurfacing flaps. Flap, especially exposed at the trunk and extremity are the best candidates for post-operative compression. From postoperative day 4, a custom-made compression garment is fitted with the aim of generating a compression pressure of 30–40 mm Hg. As a routine procedure, early compression is applied from postoperative day 5. If the flap is located at the foot, the garment is tailored from the metatarsophalangeal joint to 2.5 in. proximal from the lateral malleolus. If the flap is located at the lower leg, the garment is tailored with 2.5 in. from both the upper and lower borders of the flap. For the circumference, the garment is tailored on the basis of the contralateral circumference. The area covered by the compression garment includes the micro-anastomosis site and the flap pedicle (Fig. 12.1). Close monitoring is performed after starting mild compression with an elastic bandage for 1 day. Duration of compression starts from 2 h three times per day. Close monitoring is critical during this period. If the flap condition is reasonable, the compression is expanded to 6 h, three times per day. Ultimately, continuous compression is performed except for the sleeping time.

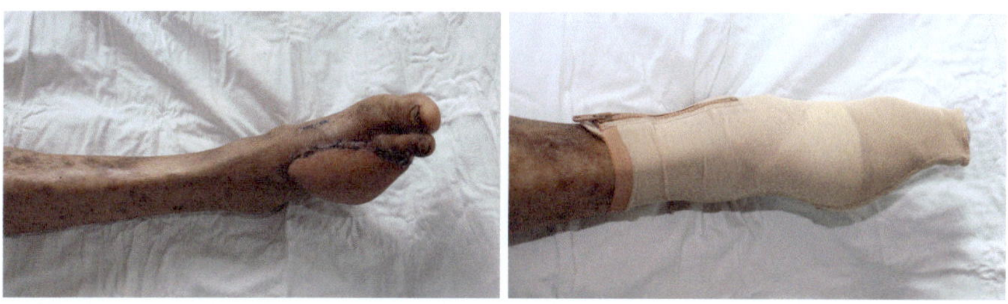

Fig. 12.1 After flap coverage surgery of diabetic ulcer on the right foot *(left)*, Compression procedure with custom-made compression garment (*right*)

12.4 Ambulation Protocol

After the compression therapy, the patients were allowed to do weight bearing after 5 days if the flap was not on the weight bearing area. When the flap was on the weight-bearing area, the partial-weight bearing was initiated after 2 weeks and full-weight bearing was starting after 6 weeks with the compression garment on.

12.5 Indicator for Delayed Compression

In case of venous congestion, we postpone the compression until the flap congestion subsides. In case of the flap with suspicious circulation, such as the flap with severe calcification of the pedicle, or with a small perforator, the compression therapy can be delayed under clinical judgment for 3~5 more days or more. As the early ambulation will be restricted in these patients, the delay is not a matter for them.

12.6 Conclusion

Early compression with 30 mm Hg customized pressure garment after flap surgery does not affect the hemodynamics of the perforator and can be safely used after extremity reconstruction before ambulation to minimize venous congestion and swelling.

References

1. Neubert N, Vogt PM, May M, et al. Does an early and aggressive combined wrapping and dangling procedure affect the clinical outcome of lower extremity free flaps?-A randomized controlled prospective study using microdialysis monitoring. J Reconstr Microsurg. 2016;32(4):262–70.
2. Chow SP, Chen DZ, Gu YD. The significance of venous drainage in free flap transfer. Plast Reconstr Surg. 1993;91(4):713–5.
3. Kolbenschlag J, Bredenbroeker P, Daigeler A, et al. Changes of oxygenation and hemoglobin-concentration in lower extremity free flaps during dangling. J Reconstr Microsurg. 2014;30(5):319–28.
4. Jokuszies A, Neubert N, Herold C, Vogt PM. Early start of the dangling procedure in lower extremity free flap reconstruction does not affect the clinical outcome. J Reconstr Microsurg. 2013;29(1):27–32.
5. Crandall CG, Shibasaki M, Yen TC. Evidence that the human cutaneous venoarteriolar response is not mediated by adrenergic mechanisms. J Physiol. 2002;538(Pt 2):599–605.
6. Ridgway EB, Kutz RH, Cooper JS, Guo L. New insight into an old paradigm: wrapping and dangling with lower-extremity free flaps. J Reconstr Microsurg. 2010;26(8):559–66.

7. D'Arpa S, Toia F, Pirrello R, Moschella F, Cordova A. Propeller flaps: a review of indications, technique, and results. Biomed Res Int. 2014;2014:986829.
8. Nelson JA, Fischer JP, Brazio PS, Kovach SJ, Rosson GD, Rad AN. A review of propeller flaps for distal lower extremity soft tissue reconstruction: is flap loss too high? Microsurgery. 2013;33(7):578–86.
9. Bekara F, Herlin C, Somda S, de Runz A, Grolleau JL, Chaput B. Free versus perforator-pedicled propeller flaps in lower extremity reconstruction: what is the safest coverage? A meta-analysis. Microsurgery. 2018;38(1):109–19.

Chapter 13
Compression for Managing Scars

Luc Téot, Marguerite Guillot Masanovic, and Christine Faure-Chazelles

Abstract Compression is one of the most powerful agent in reducing hypertrophic scars. The different modes of compression are dependant on the clinical evolution of the scar, the anatomical location and the compliance of the patient to wear uncomfortable and socially impacting therapies. This segment is in permanent challenge as most of the proposed solutions are fewly accepted by the patients, more particularly in adolescent or young adults. Since a few years new limited local technologies propose a mechanical immobilisation limited to the scar itself.

Keywords Hypertrophic scars · Keloids · Compressive therapy

13.1 Introduction

Remodeling of the newly formed extracellular matrix occurs during the final phase of normal wound healing, and starts after wound closure is completed, usually within 2–3 weeks. In a normal situation, wound épidermisation will start the down-regulation of various wound healing processes such as cell proliferation, migration and extracellular matrix synthesis and apoptosis of fibroblasts and myofibroblasts. In deep wounds, cells producing the new extracellular matrix will predominantly come from the subcutaneous fat. These cells are phenotypically different from fibroblasts issued from dermis. The collagen produced is firmer and less susceptible to degradation than the collagen usually present in skin. Linares and colleagues popularised the use of compressive garments to prevent hypertrophic scars, but compression has been used in prevention and management of scars since Ambroise Paré during the sixteenth century, Verneuil proposed compressive bandages in 1906, Blair in 1924 insisted on the influence of pressure on healing and Nason in 1942 described the role of hypoxia over the hypertrophic scarring process. At the end of the sixties Silverstein described the positive role of

L. Téot (✉) · M. G. Masanovic · C. Faure-Chazelles
Montpellier University Hospital, Montpellier Cedex, France
e-mail: l-teot@chu-montpellier.fr

R. Mani et al. (eds.), *Compression and Chronic Wound Management*,
https://doi.org/10.1007/978-3-030-01195-6_13

compressive stocking on scars located on the lower extremity. Larson observed the positive effect of collars on cervical scars [1].

13.2 Definitions

13.2.1 Hypertrophic Scars

Target scars for compression are mainly scars presenting an excessive volume.

Hypertrophy is characterized by an excessive scar proliferation which does not extend beyond the edges of the initial wound. Hypertrophic scar will usually grow for a period of time starting some months after wound closure, developing for the next 6–8 months, after which usually the progression stops and the scar gradually becomes quiescent and stabilized in terms of volume and colour. The full maturation process may take up to 2 years.

Reasons for developing scar hypertrophy remain unclear at present but cellular and message transmission dysfunction including mechanical factors are considered by the experts as the most probable contributing factor [2]. Other reasons like anatomical location, young age, origin of the wound (thermal burns particularly) and infection are recognized as contributing to a hypertrophic development.

Infected wounds are also more prone to develop hypertrophic scars with an irregular shape and a high density of collagen bundles. Persistence of inflammation over a long period of time induces a long term production of collagen from fibroblasts less likely to be submitted to the normal apoptosis process, which normally is induced as soon as the keratinocyte layers of the epidermis have been restored and wound closure is achieved. Linear hypertrophic scar (e.g. surgical/traumatic, often in the neck or shoulder regions) and wide-spreading hypertrophic scar (e.g. burns) remains within the borders of the injury. Spreading hypertrophy is usually a consequence of burns [3].

13.2.2 Keloids

Keloids are characterized by a pseudo-tumor proliferation extending over the edges of the initial wound. A keloid scar can continue to grow with time, without signs of stabilisation. It can start to develop directly after completed wound closure or could also begin growing later than a year. The pathogenesis of keloids is still unknown. Among the risk factors for keloids are genetic components, which could explain an occurence within the family but also mechanical causes [4]. Caucasians have a lower incidence of keloids than Asians and people with black skin have the highest prevalence. Young women are at highest risk and keloids often occur on multiple sites. Preferred anatomical areas for keloids are the ear lobes, the neck, the shoulder and the sternal area. Keloids are prone to recurrence after surgery.

In some countries or continents like Asia, widespread hypertrophies may resemble keloids. Still, the most important clinical criterion to differentiate between the two remains that a hypertrophic scar should be confined to the original wound margins, whereas a keloid will extend beyond the borders of the original lesion. Minor keloids appear sometimes spontaneously, on anatomical zones of mechanical traction like the thorax and the back, predominantly in dark skins. Minor keloids may stop progression or carry on their development.

Piercing may cause keloids, especially on the earlobes. No keloid has yet been described over mucosae. Major keloid is a large, raised (>0.5 cm) scar, possibly painful or pruritic and protruding into normal tissue, developing over large areas, leading to a large pending tumour, whose density and weight maybe distressful for the patient.

13.3 Mode of Action of Compression on Scars

Desmoulière et al. [5–7] confirmed the limitation in proliferation of the myofibroblats when submitted to compression. Reno et al. [8] showed that compression may act at different levels on the wound healing complex process, particularly efficient on the hypertrophy and the prurit. An increase of PGE2 was observed, as well as an increase of several growth factors and cytokins like TGF-β, TNF-α and IL1, active at the dermo-epidermic junction. An increase of the metalloproteasis 28 was also mentioned, active in the extracellular matrix, and of the TGF beta-1, a growth factor important for epithelialisation.

13.4 Compression Technologies Used in Scar Management

13.4.1 Massage and Physiotherapy

Despite the lack of clinical evidence, massage is commonly used in the treatment of (burn) scars. Nevertheless it should be used with caution because a poor indication can have side effects; it is therefore necessary to adapt the technique of massage according to the stage of the inflammation. When the inflammation has decreased, skin mobilisations can allow to improve the sliding plains of the skin and decrease adherences. Infection is a contra-indication for massage; furthermore, it is not indicated on keloids, except for the hydration part.

LPG® [9] and similar systems provide a motorised massage, applying forces combining aspiration of the skin and rolling movements.

13.4.2 Postoperative Devices Applying Compressive Forces on the Suture Edges

A better understanding of scar mechanics has been under way for several years [10] or, more recently, by applying tension to the edges through physical means (silicone sheet, "intelligent" silicone with pre-tensioning of axial fibers inserted in the matrix) [11]. Translational research has been stimulated and the optimization of mechanical devices exploiting mechanical forces has been developed, especially in the field of wound healing A recent study [12] on cadavers measured the forces of tension exerted on the edges of sutured skin and the underlying aponeurosis. These measurements can be considered as a basis for measuring the re-approximation forces of the edges in human clinical practice.

A simulation for reproducing the in vivo tension experienced by the skin, the attitude of fibroblasts from keloid scars, their matrix synthesis capacity under tension, and in vivo skin tension measured on volunteers. It has been demonstrated that the induction of tension modifies the three-dimensional model allowed expression of the genes linked to the mechanical tension of the fibroblasts. This mechanical regulation makes it possible to understand that an increased synthesis of collagen occurs in the scar when the tension is exerted strongly on the edges via the fibroblasts. The therapeutic interest of this hypothesis serves as a basis for the development of medical devices opposing edge tension (Bayat) [13].

The system using negative pressure (Prevena®) has been developed now for several years and its clinical use is under development. Several recent studies demonstrate the value of isolating the wound from any source of external contamination and of keeping it under slight tension by the foam exerting a negative pressure on the suture [14].

More recently, Parry et al. [15] proposed the *Silicone Suture Plate* (SSP) in postoperative rhytidectomies. This sterile silicone plate allowed, in a study of eight patients, to consider the scar as improved. Gurtner et al. [16] have also developed a supposed polymer medical device (Embrace®) which, after application of two booklet flaps on the scar edges, has sufficient force to keep the two scar edges in contact. This system has been tested on animals in the laboratory: it has been shown that the medical device blocked excessive tension on the edges and also blocked the profibrotic pathways of the excessive scar usually encountered in experimental and clinical situations.

In a short series, the authors used a new system based on longitudinal and transverse mechanical restriction. The originality of the system is its ability to bring the two edges together and set the skin tension. This technique gives spectacular results at the cost of a few weeks of wearing a weak allergenic adhesive based on hydrocolloids. The tension exerted on the edges after cutaneous excision surgery is a source of potential complications. Several techniques have recently been described, based on the principle of immobilizing the suture edges after surgery, and they confirm the importance of mechanical control in the prevention of pathological scars, in particular hypertrophic scars [2]. A new medical device (Zipline®) has been developed and is used clinically as a wound closure technique as an alternative to sutures in orthopedic surgery after cutaneous excision for scar revision, cutaneous tumor excision. The medical device is made up of two adhesive carboxymethylcellulose strips, which have a central reinforcing core made up of polyurethane fibers, placed on the rectilinear edges of the suture (Fig. 13.1). These strips are interconnected by tensors formed of a polyurethane thread made up of nodes which are regularly distributed along the wire and finished by collars allowing easy grasping for tensioning.

13.5 Compressive Garments

Compression should be from 24 to 32 mmHg, just above the critical capillary occlusion pressure to determine hypoxia. Several modalities can be used, alone or in association.

At the inital stage elastic or tubular bandages like Biflex*, Hypafix*, Méfix* Cohéban* (3 M) an early compression, particularly accurate on the hands. In Burns centers specialised nurses will make these temporary compressive garments at fashion, waiting for the confection of final compressive garments proposed by different companies. Interfaces like hydrocellular dressings, Medigel Z, Neopren, a synthetic rubber, silicone sheet like Cicacare* can be proposed in order to increase locally the pressure (Figs. 13.2 and 13.3).

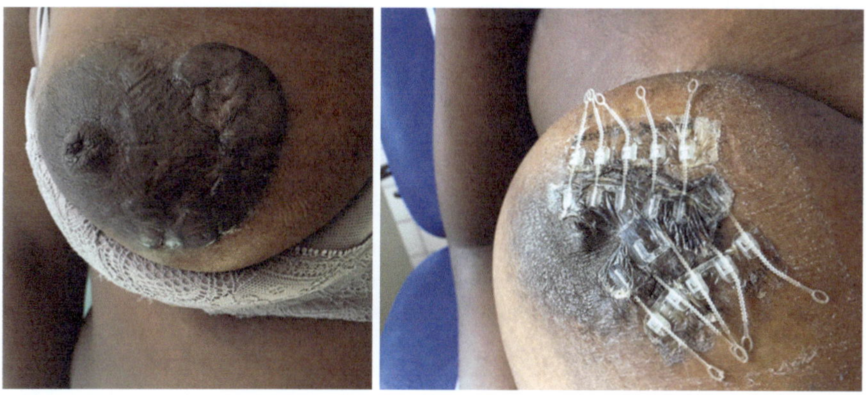

Fig. 13.1 Zipline after keloid resection

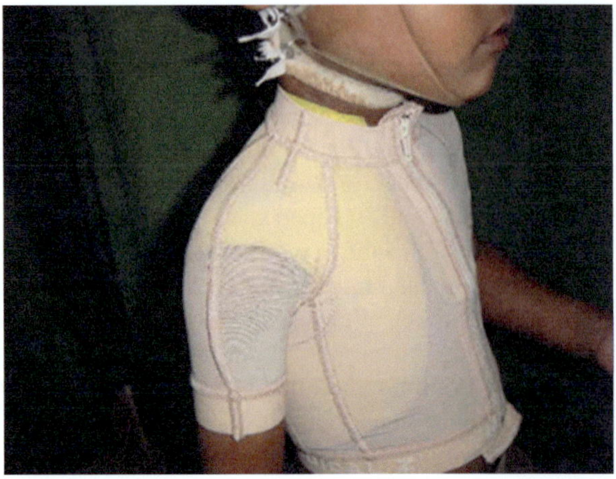

Fig. 13.2 Compressive garment plus Neopren interface

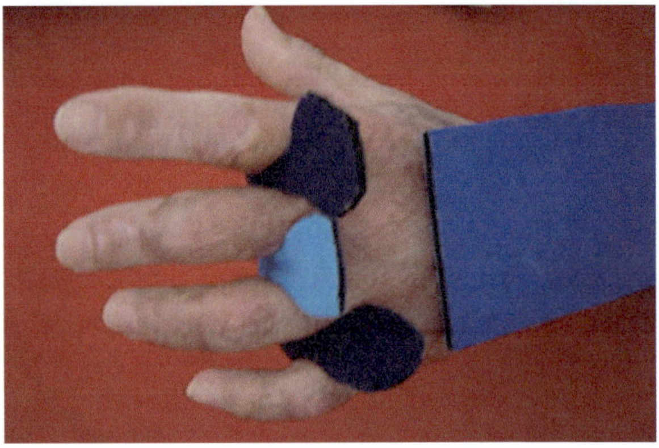

Fig. 13.3 Interdigital compressive devices

13.6 Orthotic Devices

They allow an increase of compression over a selected area, providing an anti-inflammatory effect thanks to immobilisation, they are realised with the patient maintained in position of function or maximum skin capacity in order to limit skin contractures. They are made of plaster or low température thermoplastic material at fashion, (Fig. 13.4) by a specialised professional. Masks, collars, splints for hands, or thorax (Fig. 13.5) ear compression is also more frequent due to the piercing fashion. (Figure 13.6) This has made it possible to multiply the compression strategies offered by compression garments or Orlen® plates, particularly in burn scars [17].

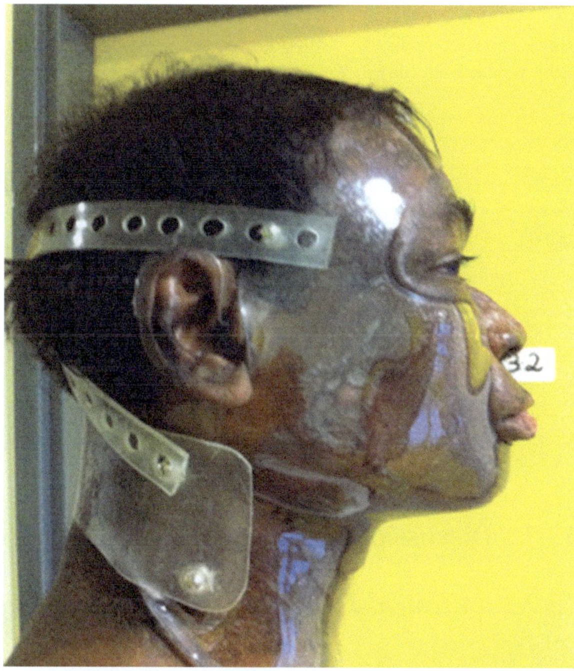

Fig. 13.4 Mask and collar in Orlen (mask and collar realised using Orlene material)

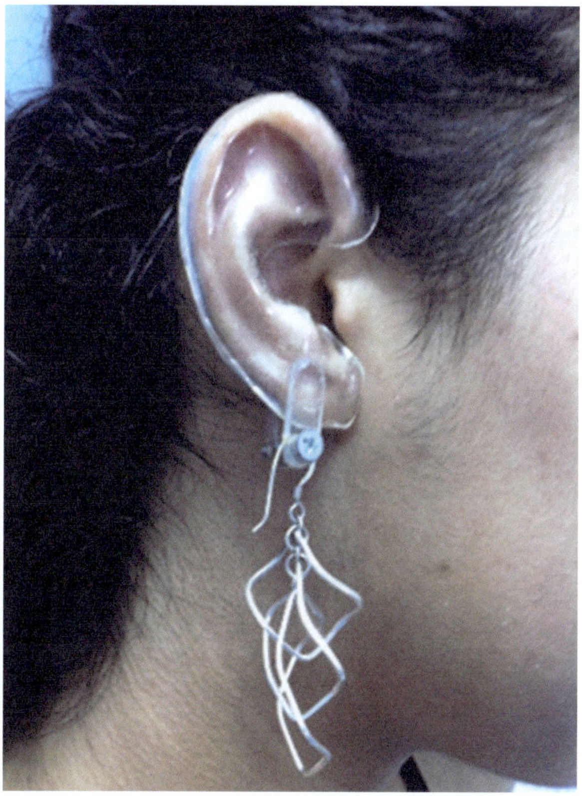

Fig. 13.5 Ear compressive device

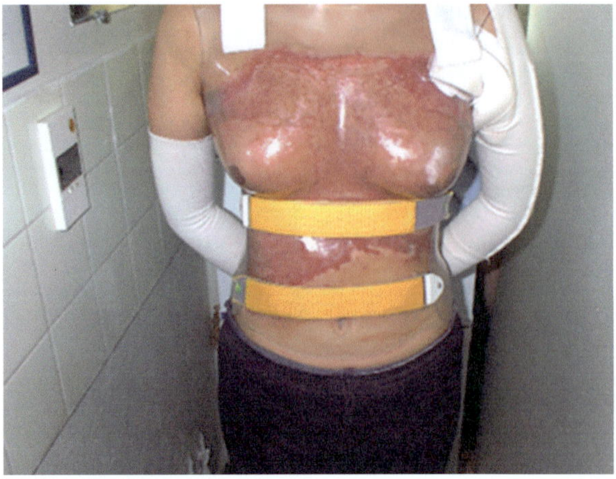

Fig. 13.6 Thoracic Orlen (thoracic device realised using Orlene material)

13.7 Discussion

13.7.1 Clinical Indications and Recommendations

Multiple articles have been published on the recommendations for the management of scars, we will only mention the most important ones. In 2002 Mustoe TA et al. [3] in their international recommendations recommend, combined with other therapeutics the use of compression for hypertrophic scars mainly in burns and prevention for keloids. In 2010 Mc Ginn CA [18] of the Rehabilitation Institute of Physical Disability of Quebec publishes an article that reflects the characteristics of the studies that were the subject of the clinical trial of Engrav et al. [19] His conclusions are that there is little evidence regarding the effectiveness of compression garments and the optimal conditions of use. Compression clothing is a therapeutic approach for which questions persist about the effectiveness. Both publications report that the use of compression garments appears to have only a minimal effect on certain aspects of the skin, thickness and stiffness and this for moderate and severe scars only.

In 2013 Atiyed BS [20] published a meta-analysis on the interest of compressive therapy for hypertrophic scars of burns, its effectiveness, its methods of application, its costs and its possible complications. Only 6 studies were selected including 316 patients, which is negligible considering the number of patients with scar tissue problems secondary to burns and the systematic prescription of compressive therapy. However, it is difficult to accurately assess the applied pressure (Laplace's law), the reduction of hypertrophy and the patient's compliance with the protocol, which is often bad because of aesthetic problems and the discomfort generated [21]. He concludes that there is no sufficient clinical evidence and that further studies are needed. In 2014 Monstrey S et al. [22] used as indications for pressotherapy (always associated with other therapeutic means)—for linear scars in prevention in subjects at risk, beyond 6 weeks and for 3 months in case of early hypertrophy and beyond 6 month if hypertrophy persists—for extended scars and prolonged healing in burns mainly, systematically in prevention, beyond 6 weeks and for 3 months in case of early hypertrophy, beyond 6 months if hypertrophy persists—for keloids of small size but especially in post-operative prevention.

In 2017 Jin-Wei Ai [23] published a review of the literature and a meta-analysis on the effectiveness of pressotherapy from 15 to 25 mmHg on hypertrophic burn scars. Twelve randomized controlled trials were included, including 710 patients with 761 hypertrophic scars. Patients receiving compressive therapy had a significant improvement in the thickness, hardness and pigmentation of hypertrophic scars across Vancouver, but more extensive and well-conducted studies would be needed to confirm these results. Conclusion: compressive therapy is part of the therapeutic arsenal for hypertrophic scars with well-codified indications in international guidelines, although the level of evidence from published studies is low, it is more of an expert consensus. However, these studies are difficult to conduct because of the difficulty of accurately assessing the degree of hypertrophy, the exact pressure applied, the patient's compliance and also difficulty in conducting randomized studies due to ethical reasons. This management involves moreover a specialized team for the preparation of orthotics, a prolonged follow-up and especially an information and adhesion of the patient to the protocol which is the most often long but also demanding, it is to say how much the patient-doctor relation is important [22]. Good compliance is essential for good clinical results.

13.8 Recommendations

Compression should be prescribed in prevention during the post op period, and worn 24 h a day. A strict check up of the skin tolerance is needed as well as a perfect adaptation of orthesis, which should be réadapte regularly. Orthesis can be worn simultaneously together with compressive garments, as long as the inflammatory process persists. The patient should be aware of the need for length and regularity in wearing the compression during more than 1 year.

References

1. Linares HA, Larson DL, Willis-Galstaun BA. Historical notes on the use of pressure in treatment of hypertrophic scars and keloids. Burns. 1993;19:17–21.
2. Bloemen MC, van der Veer WM, Ulrich MM, et al. Prevention and curative management of hypertrophic scar formation. Burns. 2009;35:463–75.
3. Mustoe TA, Cooter RD, Gold MH, Hobbs FD, Ramelet AA, Shakespeare PG, Stella M, Téot L, et al. International advisory panel on scar management. Plast Reconstr Surg. 2002;110(2):560–71.

4. Ogawa R, Okai K, Tokumura F, Mori K, Ohmori Y, Huang C, et al. The relationship between skin stretching/contraction and pathologic scarring: the important role of mechanical forces in keloid generation. Wound Repair Regen. 2012;20(2):149–57. https://doi.org/10.1111/j.1524-475X.2012.00766.x. Epub 2012 Feb 14
5. Desmoulière A, Geinoz A, Gabbiani F, Gabbiani G. Transforming growth factor-beta 1 induces alpha-smooth muscle actin expression in granulation tissue myofibroblasts and in quiescent and growing cultured fibroblasts. J Cell Biol. 1993;122(1):103–11.
6. Desmouliere A, Badid C, Bochaton-Piallat ML, Gabbiani G. Apoptosis during wound healing, fibrocontractive diseases and vascular wall injury. Int J Biochem Cell Biol. 1997;29(1):19–30.
7. Darby IA, Laverdet B, Bonté F, Desmoulière A. Fibroblasts and myofibroblasts in wound healing. Clin Cosmet Investig Dermatol. 2014;7:301–11.
8. Renò F, Sabbatini M, Lombardi F, et al. In vitro mechanical compression induces apoptosis and regulates cytokines release in hypertrophic scars. Wound Repair Regen. 2003;11:331–6.
9. Gavroy JP, Dinard J, Costagliola M, Rouge D, Griffe O, Téot L, Ster F. LPG and the cutaneous softening of burns. J Plaies et Cicatrisation Dec. 1996;5:42–6.
10. Harn HI, Ogawa R, Hsu CK, Hughes MW, Tang MJ, Chuong CM. The tension biology of wound healing. Exp Dermatol. 2017. https://doi.org/10.1111/exd.13460. [Epub ahead of print] Review.
11. Longaker MT, Rohrich RJ, Greenberg L, Furnas H, Wald R, Bansal V, et al. A randomized controlled trial of the embrace advanced scar therapy device to reduce incisional scar formation. Plast Reconstr Surg. 2014;134(3):536–46.
12. Hwang K, Kim HJ, Kim KY, Han SH, Hwang SJ. Skin tension related to tension reduction sutures. Adv Wound Care (New Rochelle). 2014;3(10):626–34.
13. Suarez E, Syed F, Rasgado TA, Walmsley A, Mandal P, Bayat A. Skin equivalent tensional forces alters keloid fibroblast behavior and phenotype. Aesthetic Plast Surg. 2014;38:767–78.
14. Kilpadi DV, Lessing C, Derrick K. Healed porcine incisions previously treated with a surgical incision management system: mechanical, histomorphometric, and gene expression properties. Biophys J. 2014;106(4):932–43. https://doi.org/10.1016/j.bpj.2013.12.002.
15. Parry JR, Stupak HD, Johnson CM. The immediate use of a silicone sheet wound closure device in scar reduction and prevention. Ear Nose Throat J. 2016;95(2):E27–33.
16. Barnes LA, Marshall CD, Leavitt T, Hu MS, Moore AL, Gonzalez JG, Longaker MT, Gurtner GC. Mechanical forces in cutaneous wound healing: emerging therapies to minimize scar formation. Adv Wound Care (New Rochelle). 2018;7(2):47–56. https://doi.org/10.1089/wound.2016.0709. Review
17. Roques C. Pressure therapy to treat burn scars. Wound Repair Regen. 2002;10(2):122–5.
18. Mc Ginn CA, Boucher N. Institut de Réadaptation en déficience Physique de Québec. Les vêtements compressifs dans le traitement et la réadaptation des grands Brûlés. Exploration préliminaire de la littérature; 2010.
19. Engrav LH, Heimbach DH, Rivara FP, et al. 12-year within-wound study of the effectiveness of pressure garment therapy. Burns. 2010;36:975–83.
20. Atiyeh BS. Nonsurgical management of hypertrophic scars: evidence-based therapies, standard practices, and emerging methods. Aesthet Plast Surg. 2007;31:468–92.
21. Ripper S, Renneberg B, Landmann C, et al. Adherence to pressure garment therapy in adult burn patients. Burns. 2009;35:657–64.
22. Monstrey S, Middelkoop E, Vranckx JJ, Bassetto F, Ziegler UE, Meaume S, Téot L. Updated scar management practical guidelines: non-invasive and invasive measures. J Plast Reconstr Aesthet Surg. 2014;67:1017–25.
23. Jin-Wei AI, Liu J-t, Pei S-D, Liu Y, Li D-S, Lin H-M, Pei B. The effectiveness of pressure therapy (15–25 mmHg) for hypertrophic burn scars: a systematic review and meta-analysis. Sci Rep. 2017;7:40185.

Appendix

3M (UK)

- Address: 3M Centre, Cain Road, Bracknell, RG12 8HT, UK
- Customer Service number (UK): +44 (0) 870 536 0036
- Website: https://www.3m.co.uk/3M/en_GB/company-uk/

Compression bandages

- Single-layer bandages

Coban Self-Adherent Wrap

- Multi-layer bandages

Coban 2 Compression System
Coban 2 Compression System Kit
Coban 2 Lite Compression System
Coban 2 Lite Compression System Kit
ArjoHuntleigh (UK)

- Address: Arjo House, Houghton Hall Business Park, Houghton Regis, Beds, LU5 5XF, UK
- Customer Service number (UK): +44 (0) 158 274 5700
- Website: https://www.arjo.com/en-gb/

Compression devices

- Intermittent pneumatic compression
- **Flowtron**

Aspen Medical Europe Ltd (UK)

- Address: Aspen Medical Europe Ltd, Clinitron House, Ashby House, Ashby Park, Ashby de la Zouch, Leicestershire, LE65 1JG, UK
- Customer Service number (UK): +44 (0) 153 041 1000

R. Mani et al. (eds.), *Compression and Chronic Wound Management*,
https://doi.org/10.1007/978-3-030-01195-6

- Email: customers@aspenmedicaleurope.com
- Website: http://www.aspenmedicaleurope.com

Compression hosiery

- Multi-layer hosiery

- **AndoFlex TLC XL with Malodour Control 2 Layer Kit**
- **AndoFlex UBZ 2 Layer Kit with Zinc**
- **AndoFlex TLC Lite with Malodour Control 10cm 2 Layer Kit**
- **AndoFlex TLC with Malodour Control 10cm 2 Layer Kit**

Bastos Viegas S.A. (Portugal)

- Address: Bastos Viegas, S.A, Avenida da Fábrica 298, 4560-164 Guilhufe, Penafiel, Portugal
- Customer Service number (Por): +351 255 729 500
- Email: geral@bastosviegas.com
- Website: http://www.bastosviegas.com/index.php

Compression hosiery

- Single-layer hosiery

Tubular Support Bandages 4214
Bauerfeind AG (Germany)

- Address: Bauerfiend AG, Triebeser Straße 16, 07937 Zeulenroda-Triebes, Germany
- Customer Service number (Ger): +49 (0) 36628 66 1000
- Website: https://www.bauerfeind.de/en/home.html

Compression hosiery

- Multi-layer hosiery

- **Ulcertec**

BSN medical Limited (UK)

- Address: BSN medical Limited, Block C Willerby Hill Business Park, Willerby, Hull, East Yorkshire, HU10 6FE, UK
- Customer Service number (UK): +44 (0) 148 267 0100
- Email: orders.uk@bsnmedical.com
- Website (UK): https://www.bsnmedical.co.uk

Compression bandages

- Single-layer bandages

- **Compralin**
- **Tensopress**
- Multi-layer bandages

Jobst Compri2
Jobst Compri2 Lite
Jobst Comprifore
Jobst Comprifore Latex-free
Jobst Comprifore Lite
Jobst Comprifore Lite Latex-free
Compression hosiery

- Multi-layer hosiery

- **Jobst UlcerCare**
- **Jobst UlcerCare Custom Fit**

Compression devices

- Adjustable compression systems

- **Jobst Farrow Wrap**

Cardinal Health (USA):

- Address: Cardinal Health, 7000 Cardinal Place, Dublin, OH 43017, USA
- Customer Service number: +1 800 964 5227
- Website: https://www.cardinalhealth.com/en.html

Compression devices

- Intermittent pneumatic compression

- **Kendal SCD**

CliniSupplies Healthcare Solutions (UK)

- Address: CliniSupplies, Qualitas House, 100 Elmgrove Road, Harrow, HA1 2RW
- Customer Service number (UK): +44 (0) 208 863 4168
- Email: info@clinisupplies.co.uk
- Website: https://www.clinisupplies.co.uk/

Compression hosiery

- Multi-layer hosiery

- **Clini Duo40**

ConvaTec (UK)

- Address: Customer Services, ConvaTec Ltd, Unit 20, First Avenue, Deeside Industrial Park, Deeside, Flintshire, CH5 2NU, UK
- Customer Service number (UK): +44 (0) 124 428 4882
- Email: uk.customerservice@convatec.com
- Website: https://www.convatec.co.uk/

Compression bandages

- Single-layer bandages
- **Surepress**

Credenhill (UK)

- Address: Credenhill Limited, 10 Cossall Industrial Estate, Ilkeston, Derbyshire, DE7 5UG, UK
- Customer Service number (UK): +44 (0) 115 932 0144
- Email: sales@credenhill.co.uk
- Website: http://www.credenhill.co.uk/

Compression hosiery

- Single-layer hosiery
- **Credalast**
- **Venosan 2000**
- **Venosan Legline**
- Multi-layer hosiery
- **Venosan 8000 Ulcerfit**

Firstkind Limited (UK)

- Address: Firstkind Limited, Hawk House, Gomm Road, High Wycombe HP13 7DL, UK
- Customer Service number (UK): +44 (0) 845 222 2921
- Email: geko.support@fistkindmedical.com
- Website: http://www.gekodevices.com/en-uk/

Compression devices

- Powered muscle stimulators
- **Geko**

FlowAid (USA)

- Address: FlowAid Medical Technologies Corporation, 44 Wall Street, 2nd Floor, New York, NY 10005, USA
- Customer Service number (USA): +1 212 461 3225
- Email: info@flowaid.com
- Website: http://flowaid.com/

Compression devices

- Sequential compression devices:

FlowAid
Haddenham Healthcare (UK)

- Address: Haddenham Healthcare, Crendon House, Long Crendon Industrial Park, Long Crendon, HP18 9BB, UK
- Customer Service number (UK): +44 (0) 184 420 8842

- Email: sales@hadhealth.com
- Website: https://hadhealth.com/

Compression bandages

- Single-layer bandages

Clinistretch Short

- Multi-layer bandages
- **Clinistretch**
- Padding
- **Clinistretch Soft**
- Compression devices
- Adjustable Velcro wraps
- **Haddenham Easywrap**

H&R Healthcare (UK) - (some products manufactured by Carolon Company)

- Address (UK): H&R Healthcare Ltd, 3 Redcliff Road, Melton Park, Melton, Hull, HU14 3RS, UK
- Customer Service number (UK): +44 (0) 148 263 1606
- Email: info@hrhealthcare.co.uk
- Website (UK): http://hrhealthcare.co.uk/

Compression bandages

- Multi-layer bandages
- **Hero H-2**
- Compression hosiery
- Single-layer hosiery
- **Carolon Multi-layer Compression System Understocking Pack**
- Multi-layer hosiery
- **Carolon Multi-layer Compression System**

Compression devices

- Sub-bandage pressure monitors

Carolon Smart Sleeve
Jobskin (UK)

- Address: Jobskin, Unit 13a Harrington Mill, Leopold St, Long Eaton, Nottingham NG10 4QG, UK
- Customer Service number (UK): +44 (0) 115 973 4300
- Email: orders@jobskin.co.uk
- Website: https://www.jobskin.co.uk/

Compression hosiery

- Single-layer hosiery
- **Premier MTM Ulcer Care Sock**
- Multi-layer hosiery
- **Alleviant Ulcer Care Kit**

Lohmann & Rauscher (Germany)

– Address: Lohmann & Rauscher GmbH & Co. KG, Irlicher Straße 55, DE-56567 Neuwied, Germany
– Customer Service number (Ger): +49 2634 99-0
– Email: info@de.LRmed.com
– Website: https://www.lohmann-rauscher.com/en/

Compression bandages

- Single-layer bandages

Atico
Rosidal K

- Multi-layer bandages

Atico 2C
Rosidal TCS

- Padding
- **Cellona Undercast**
- **FlexiBan**
- **Rosidal Soft**
- Compression hosiery
- Single-layer hosiery
- **ActiLymph Hosiery Kit**
- **Activa British Standard Compression Hosiery**
- **Activa Class 1 Unisex Sock**
- **Activa Class 2 Unisex Sock**
- Multi-layer hosiery

Activa Leg Ulcer Hosiery Kits
Compression devicies

- Adjustable compression systems

ReadyWrap
medi UK Limited (UK – part of medi Group)

– Address: medi UK Limited, Plough Lane, Hereford, HR4 0EL, UK
– Customer Service number (UK): +44 (0) 143 237 3500
– Email: enquiries@mediuk.co.uk
– Website: https://www.mediuk.co.uk/

Compression hosiery

- Single-layer hosiery

- **Duomed Soft – BS Hosiery (medi UK)**
- Multi-layer hosiery
- **Medivan ulcer kit (medi UK)**
- Compression devices
- Adjustable Velcro wraps
- **Juxtacures (medi UK)**
- **Juxtalite (medi UK) – also known as CircAid**
- Sub-bandage pressure monitors
- **PicoPress (medi Australia)**
- **Kikuhime (medi Australia)**
- Adjustable compression systems

Juxtacures
Juxtalite – also known as CircAid
Mölnlycke Health Care AB (Sweden)

- Address: Gamlestadsvägen 3C, 415 02 Göteborg, Sweden
- Customer Service number (Swe): +46 31 722 30 00
- Website: https://www.molnlycke.co.uk/

Compression bandages

- Single-layer bandages

- **Setopress**

Otivio AS (Norway)

- Address: Otivio AS, Gaustadalléen 2, N-0349 Oslo, Norway
- Customer Service number (USA): +47 468 90 416
- Email: info@otivio.com
- Website: https://www.otivio.com/

Compression devices

- Intermittent pneumatic compression

FlowOx™
Robinson Healthcare (UK)

- Address: Robinson Healthcare Limited, Lawn Road., Carlton-in-Lindrick, Worksop, S81 9LB, UK
- Customer Service number (UK): +44 (0) 190 973 5000
- Email: orders@robinsonhealthcare.com
- Website: http://www.robinsonhealthcare.com/

Compression bandages

- Multi-layer bandages

- **Ultra Four**

Sallis Healthcare (UK)

- Address: Sallis Healthcare, Vernon Works, Waterford Street, Basford, Nottingham, NG6 0DH, UK
- Customer Service number (UK): +44 (0) 115 978 7841
- Email: info@sallis.co.uk
- Website: http://sallis.co.uk/

Compression hosiery

- Single-layer hosiery

Eesilite
Sigvaris (Switzerland)

- Address: Sigvaris Management AG, St. Georgenstrasse 70, 8401 Winterthur, Switzerland
- Customer Service number (Swi): Tel.: +41 52 265 00 00
- Website: https://www.sigvaris.com/global/en

Compression hosiery

- Multi-layer hosiery

- **Ulcer X Kit and Ulcer X Liners**

Smith & Nephew plc (UK & Ireland)

- Address: Smith & Nephew, Croxley Park, Building 5, Hatters Lane, Watford, Hertfordshire, WD18 8YE, UK
- Customer Service number (UK): +44 (0) 800 015 7573
- Email: customer.services.uki@smith-nephew.com
- Website: http://www.smith-nephew.com/

Compression bandages

- Multi-layer bandages

- **Profore**
- **Profore Lite**
- **Profore Latex Free**
- **Profore Latex Free Lite**

Synergy Health plc (UK)

- Address: Synergy Health plc, Ground Floor Stella, Windmill Hill Business Park, Whitehill Way, Swindon, SN5 6NX, UK
- Customer Service number (UK): +44 (0) 179 360 1000

- Email: assistance@synergyhealthplc.com
- Website: https://www.synergyhealthplc.com/en

Compression hosiery

- Multi-layer hosiery
- **Compression Leg Ulcer Kit**

Talley Group (UK)

- Address: Talley Group Limited, Abbey Park Industril Estate, Premier Way, Romsey, Hampshire, SO51 9DQ, UK
- Customer Service number (UK): +44 (0)1794 503500
- Email: exportsales@talleygroup.com
- Website: http://www.talleygroup.com/

Compression devices

- Intermittent compression devices

Synchro system
TTP Ventus

- Address: TTP Ventus, Melbourn Science Park, Melbourn, Hertfordshire, SG8 6EE, UK
- Customer Service number (UK): +44 (0)1763 262626
- Email: enquiries@ttpventus.com
- Website: https://www.ttpventus.com/

Compression devices

- Intermittent pneumatic compression
- **Ventus Disc Pump System**

Urgo Medical

- Address: Urgo Limited, Sullington Road, Shepshed, Loughborough, Leicestershire, UK
- Customer Service number (UK): +44 (0) 150 950 2051
- Email: woundcare@uk.urgo.com
- Website: www.urgo.co.uk

Compression bandages

- Single-layer bandages
- **K-Plus**
- **K-ThreeC**
- **Ko-Flex**
- Multi-layer bandages
- **K-Four**
- **UrgoKTwo**

- **UrgoKTwo Reduced**
- **UrgoKTwo with UrgoStart**
- Padding
- **K-Soft**
- Compression hosiery
- Single-layer hosiery

- **Altiform British Standard Compression Hosiery**
- **Altiform British Standard Made to Measure Compression Hosiery**

AltiMed (UK – part of URGO medical group)

- Address: AltiMed, Sullington Road, Shepshed, Loughborough, Leicestershire, LE12 9JG, UK
- Customer Service number (UK): +44 1509 510720
- Email: enquiries@altimed.co.uk
- Website: http://www.altimed.co.uk/

Compression hosiery

- Multi-layer hosiery

- **Altipress 40 Leg Ulcer Kit**
- **Altipress 40 Made to Measure Ulcer Kit**

Index

R. Mani et al. (eds.), *Compression and Chronic Wound Management*,
https://doi.org/10.1007/978-3-030-01195-6

MIX
Papier aus verantwortungsvollen Quellen
Paper from responsible sources
FSC® C105338

If you have any concerns about our products,
you can contact us on
ProductSafety@springernature.com

In case Publisher is established outside the EU,
the EU authorized representative is:
Springer Nature Customer Service Center GmbH
Europaplatz 3, 69115 Heidelberg, Germany

Printed by Libri Plureos GmbH
in Hamburg, Germany